UNDERSTANDING
BRAIN and MIND
A CONNECTIONIST PERSPECTIVE

UNDERSTANDING
BRAIN and MIND
A CONNECTIONIST PERSPECTIVE

YEHUDA SALU
Howard University, USA

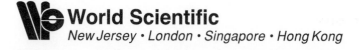
World Scientific
New Jersey • London • Singapore • Hong Kong

Published by

World Scientific Publishing Co. Pte. Ltd.

P O Box 128, Farrer Road, Singapore 912805

USA office: Suite 1B, 1060 Main Street, River Edge, NJ 07661

UK office: 57 Shelton Street, Covent Garden, London WC2H 9HE

British Library Cataloguing-in-Publication Data
A catalogue record for this book is available from the British Library.

UNDERSTANDING BRAIN AND MIND
A Connectionist Perspective

ISBN 981-02-4792-3
ISBN 981-02-4795-8 (pbk)

Printed in Singapore.

To Pnina, Eran, and Gil

Contents

PREFACE

Connectionism is a scientific discipline that deals with the relationships between properties of individual neurons, the connections between them, and the overall performances of the neural networks that they form. It has two major interdependent divisions: one dealing with biological and the other with artificial neural networks. When dealing with biological neural networks, connectionism provides tools for integrating known separate biological facts into comprehensive descriptions of systems. Connectionism also helps in the evaluation of hypothetical mechanisms that might explain observed behaviors of entire systems. When dealing with artificial neural networks, connectionism helps in the design of artificial-intelligence means that perform specified tasks. The operation rules of the neurons and of the connections that are used by those artificial neural networks are more flexible, compared to biological ones. However, artificial neural networks retain some semblance of biological neural networks.

In connectionist models, neurons are represented by nodes and connections between neurons are represented by links. Each particular connectionist model determines which biological features are exactly duplicated by the nodes and the links, which are approximated, and which are ignored. Models may also assign to their nodes features that are not possessed by neurons. All the assigned features determine how the network of nodes would handle information. The goal of the designer of a biological model is to select the features so that the system, as a whole, would execute certain operations in a way that reproduces observed macroscopic behaviors of the simulated biological system. Models of biological networks can be implemented in practical artificial-intelligence applications.

This book introduces a connectionist model that deals with operations of the brain. It relates principles of neural operation, network architecture, data processing principles, and macroscopic observable behavior of the system. As a connectionist model, it consists of nodes that are connected by links. The nodes have some similarity to neurons, and the links are similar to the connection between neurons.

Currently, a one-to-one detailed mapping of all the neurons of a brain, or even of major parts of them, onto nodes of a connectionist network is not feasible. There are too many neurons and synapses, and too many anatomical and physiological details are not known. To bypass these obstacles, connectionist models rely on small numbers of nodes, relative to the numbers of neurons in biological systems. A node usually represents a large number of neurons, and a link represents a large number of synaptic connections. The models rely on robust biological features that are deemed the most important. Nodes and links may also have performance features that so far have not been found in single neurons. The rationale for including these features is that they may be performed in the brain by groups of other neurons, and affect the neuron that is represented by the node. For the moment, the detailed biological mechanisms behind these features are beyond the scope of the connectionist model. With all these inevitable limitations, connectionist models can provide general understanding of processes that may take place in the brain and affect behavior. The models can integrate isolated facts from various scientific disciplines, including biology, psychology, and computer science, into coherent descriptions of the system.

There have been many connectionist models describing various aspects of the operation of the brain and of its sub-systems. The model presented here combines basic ideas that have been used in different models with ideas that are probably unique to the model. Two of the latter, which are motivated by biological observations, are the concepts of 'arena' and 'pixel's-cluster'.

An arena is a group of organized nodes that can represent external events. The innate organization of the arena is akin to implicit knowledge of the system. For example, retinal neurons can represent external events, such as two objects that we see. Two retinal images that are apart from each other are caused by objects that are also apart from each other. The system can tell that the objects are apart because of the physical structure of eye and the organization of the neurons of the retina.

Each arena has detectors, which analyze the information that the arena displays, and projectors, which create in the arena simulations of events. Projected events are processed by the detectors of the arena, and are important in various thinking processes.

A pixel's-cluster is an element of the model that imitates the columnar organization of the cortex. Similar to neurons in a cortical column, which represent various properties of an element of an object, arenas in the model have pixel's-clusters, each of which representing various properties of a corresponding external pixel.

Uncovering biological processes at the synaptic level is experimentally very challenging, especially when the processes have to be correlated with macroscopic behaviors of the entire organism. This model explains a number of observed macroscopic behaviors of the system based on a limited number of synaptic processes. The model assumes that these processes are controlled by specialized nodes. Thus, the model uses two types of nodes: those that represent the information that the brain has to store and to use, and those that control the handling of that information. In the brain, controlling the use of information may be carried out by specialized neurons, but it may be also carried out by entire networks or by parts of neurons. Once these processes are uncovered, they could be implemented in the model.

In general, the model presented here is based on very general operation principles of single neurons and on observed organizational and operational characteristics of the mind and the nervous system. It illustrates how the same basic data representation and data processing principles apply to simple processes and to very complex ones. The model does not describe all the possible macroscopic activities of the brain, but it is hoped that the perspective that it provides should help in developing models for those activities. Since many biological observations were obtained from a variety of animals, sub-systems of the model are also applicable to non-human systems.

The model treats the brain as a system that receives, stores, manipulates, and transmits data. It employs a fundamental scheme of encoding and processing data and illustrates how general observed behaviors of brain and mind emerge from those fundamental principles.

The brain is a dynamic system, and any brain model must be able to represent dynamic processes. This property of a model is referred to in the following as 'simulating' the activity of the brain, which is carried out by a 'simulation program'.

The model provides a framework for computer programs and applications that simulate various aspects of brain operations. The elements of a program, such as the nature of the participating neurons, how they are organized into networks, and the external conditions are to be provided by the user. The implemented program could then simulate the behavior of the system for the given situation.

The material is presented in three partially overlapping cycles that start with general descriptions and then focus on details. The chapters of the first cycle describe how the elements of the model relate to neurons and to components of computers. They emphasize what are the main similarities and what are the most significant differences between nodes on one hand and biological neurons and computer memory cells and other computer components on the other hand. Then, the main ideas that the model borrows from computer science, in particular strategies of data storage and management, are introduced. The second cycle of the presentation describes in broad terms how the model represents a variety of brain operations, including pattern analysis, data storage and retrieval, and basic thinking patterns. The third cycle introduces the precise specifications of the elements of the model and the operation rules that it uses. This is done in a way that should make it possible to write computer implementations of the model for particular biological or artificial situations. Examples of how some advanced processes can be represented by fundamental ones are detailed. The third cycle concludes with an illustration of how the model can treat complex conscious and unconscious mental activities.

1. NODES AND NEURAL NETWORKS

Representing existence and presence

Neurons and nodes

Neurons are the major building blocks of the brain. Approximately 10^{13} neurons make up the human brain, and they come in a variety of shapes and sizes. Many models of neural networks have been developed for explaining the function of different parts of the brain. Most of these models rely on what may be called 'standard neurons', which are assumed to encompass the most important properties that are common to biological neurons.

A standard neuron (figure 1.1) has three main parts: input channels, body, and output channels. The input channels represent the dendrites of biological neurons. The body represents the soma, and the output channels represent the axon and the axonic branches. Standard neurons are connected to each other by synapses. A synapse connects an output channel of one neuron to an input channel of another.

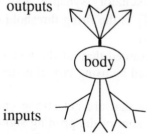

Figure 1.1: Schematics of the main parts of a standard neuron. Inputs (dendrites), body (soma), and outputs (axonic tree).

Input signals that enter the neuron in the form of electrical pulses reach the body of the neuron. There they are added, and build up the potential across the membrane of the body. Once that potential passes a certain threshold, the neuron sends out trains of electric pulses, through the branches of the axonic tree. This is called firing. In some neurons, the frequency of the output pulses is proportional to the potential of the body. Standard neurons can simulate these activity-states with different resolution levels. The least refined representation is by a binary neuron. It has two distinct states: quiet and firing. In more refined representations, a standard neuron can fire at a variety of intensities, which correspond to the frequencies of the output pulses. Some models assign significance to the temporal firing patterns of their neurons, while others do not consider that feature.

The same output signals are sent through all the output channels of a firing neuron. As a signal passes from a firing neuron through a synapse to a receiving neuron, its intensity is regulated by the synaptic weight. Different output channels of the same neuron may have different synaptic weights.

Like neurons in neural networks, the nodes of the connectionist model have two states: firing and quiet. Connections between nodes have synaptic weights. The architecture of the network and the synaptic weights determine how information flows in the connectionist model.

Like a neuron, a node fires when the sum of its weighted inputs is greater than its firing threshold, as expressed by the relationship:

$$\sum_i A_i \cdot \sigma_{ij} \geq T_j \qquad\qquad [1.1]$$

Where A_i indicates the input to synapse i (zero or one for input coming from a binary node); σ_{ij} is the synaptic weight from node i to node j (A positive synaptic weight means excitatory synapse, and a negative weight means inhibitory synapse.); and T_j is the firing threshold of node j (will be assumed one for all the nodes here).

In the following, it will be assumed that all the nodes are binary. Non-binary properties will be represented by using virtual nodes, to be introduced soon.

A node that gets input signals that are not strong enough to cause its firing is said to be **primed**. If the sum of the priming signals is greater than zero, it will take less additional inputs to activate that primed node. If that sum is negative, due to negative (inhibitory) weights leading to it, stronger additional signals will be required to activate that node.

Neurons can be divided into three main groups: (1) Input neurons, which are stimulated by external causes such as light or concentration of sugar in the blood. These neurons have specialized sensors that convert the external stimuli into electrical signals that propagate to the neuron. (2) Output neurons, which stimulate external units such as muscles or glands. These neurons are connected to non-neuronal elements, and activate them by signals transmitted through the axonal connections. (3) Inner neurons, which are all the neurons in-between the input and the output neurons. In addition to information that flows in the input-inner-output direction, input neurons may also be affected by signals that they receive from the network, and output neurons may send signals to neurons in the network. Neurons may communicate with each other not only through connecting synapses, but also by eliciting the release of chemicals that propagate in the surroundings of the network and affect the activity of other neurons. Connectionist models can simulate these processes by regular input and output channels of nodes.

A correspondence was found between the external stimulation of various areas of the body and the firing of neurons in the somatosensory cortex. These firing neurons may be considered as the internal representations of the corresponding external events. Similarly, the stimulation of certain neurons in the motor cortex elicits the activity of well-correlated muscle groups. Thus, these firing neurons may be considered the representations of their corresponding muscular activities. Activities of other cortical neurons have been correlated with specific external stimuli. For example, certain neurons in the visual cortex fire when linear objects of certain spatial orientation are present at certain points of the field of view. Other neurons fire when a face appears in the field of view. Such neurons may be considered as the representations of their corresponding concepts.

This idea is extended to a general hypothesis, stating that any event or concept that the brain handles is represented by its own neuron. The existence of the concept in the system is represented by the existence of the neuron in the network. The system handles concepts that are represented by neurons. The firing of a neuron indicates that its concept is present in the current scenario, which is being handled by the system. This idea is dubbed as 'the grandmother-neuron hypothesis'. It means that any concept that the brain can handle, such as grandmother, is represented by its own neuron. When that concept is present in the ongoing happening, the neuron fires.

Connectionist models simulate the brain as a network of nodes, in which signals propagate between connected nodes. The degree by which nodes of a model replicate the activities of biological neurons varies from model to model. However, in all models, the connections between the nodes determine the flow of the signals in the network, and the characteristics of individual nodes determine the conditions for their firing. In such models, firing nodes represent the various aspects of presence that the body experiences: A firing sensory node represents the presence of the particular external event that has caused its firing. A firing motor node represents the presence of the activity of the activated body part. The firing of an intermediate node represents the presence of the pattern of firing nodes by which it has been activated, or the presence of internal processes. A quiet network stores the passive properties of the network. These properties determine how the network would react to external stimuli, and how it would function when its inner nodes are the source of the activity.

In all models, the synaptic weights between the nodes (or between neurons) determine the flow of activation in the network. The weights thus determine which nodes will activate which, or in other words, how the presence of some concepts depends on the presence of others. This is the type of information that networks can express, and they encode this information by their synaptic weights.

Virtual nodes

Although experimental evidence indicates that correlation does exist between some external events and firing of certain neurons, the correlation may not be one to one. Neurons that fire when grandmother appears in sight may be non-specific to grandmother. Each of them may also fire when some other objects appear. It is reasonable to assume that the appearance of grandmother causes the firing of a pattern of neurons that, as a pattern, are unique to grandmother. If that is the case, such a pattern may be represented by a single virtual node, whose firing represents the presence of grandmother. A virtual node is a regular node that does not have a corresponding unique neuron in the system. A model may declare and use virtual nodes at its own discretion. An outside observer cannot tell whether an information entity is represented by a real or by a virtual node, based solely on the performance of the system. For example, if grandmother, grandfather, and uncle are distinct concepts that the system recognizes, they may be represented by combination of the real nodes A, B, and C as follows:

'grandmother' = (A&B), 'grandfather' = (B&C), and 'uncle' = (A&C). None of these concepts is represented by a unique node. However, the combination (A&B) can be represented by a virtual node, which would represent the concept 'grandmother'. Similarly, 'grandfather' and 'uncle' may be represented by their virtual nodes.

When a group of firing nodes cause the activation of another node, it can be said that the latter represents the entire group. A group of firing nodes that do not cause the firing of any other node can be represented in the model by a virtual node.

Events that happen along some time interval are represented in the brain by a corresponding sequence of firing neurons. Virtual nodes can represent concepts whose constituting neurons or nodes fire concurrently or sequentially in time.

Firing of neurons is a main staple in the functioning of the brain. However, there are important neural processes, which are related to information processing, that are carried out by other biological mechanisms. For example, changing of synaptic weights, which is believed to be the brain mechanism for recording information, may depend on firing of neurons, but it is not firing per-se. Such mechanisms may be included as concepts in brain models, and as concepts, they would be represented by virtual nodes. For example, a brain model may have a virtual node that represents the concept of 'increase synaptic weight between any two firing nodes'. When this virtual node is activated by other firing nodes, the simulation program will make the appropriate synaptic weight changes. Such a virtual node exists only in the model of the brain, not in the brain itself. It has all the properties of a real node, and its purpose is to facilitate the description of the events that occur in the brain.

Each virtual node of the types described so far is representing a number of neurons or nodes. In one type of virtual nodes, this situation is reversed: A number of virtual nodes is used to represent one neuron. A neuron may fire in various frequencies and temporal patterns. In some cases, the rate of firing of a neuron is proportional to the potential of its body, which depends on the intensity of the input. Thus, the firing frequency of one neuron can encode a variety of input patterns. It might be simpler to break up the output of the neuron into segments, each of which representing just one input pattern. To accomplish this goal, a neuron that has a range of possible firing frequencies will be replaced by a group of virtual binary nodes. Each of these virtual nodes will represent a different segment of firing frequencies. Such a group of virtual nodes is mutually exclusive to each other–no more than one of them can fire at the same time.

Commissioned and non-commissioned nodes

The innate brain is wired to represent certain external and internal events. When those events happen, their corresponding neurons fire–thus representing the presence of the events. There are indications that new neurons are not generated in the brain after a certain point at a very young age. The implication of this is that as the brain learns its environment, its innate connections are modified in order to represent the various aspects of the learned events. It is not known if a certain number of the neurons of the innate brain are commissioned to represent particular concepts, and all the other neurons are non-commissioned (blank). If each concept is represented by a unique neuron (the grandmother hypothesis), the brain must have commissioned and non-commissioned neurons. Non-commissioned neurons can then be recruited to represent new concepts. The model presented here avoids the issue of the biological significance of 'grandmother neurons' by allowing the use of virtual nodes. By so doing, the model neither endorses nor rejects that hypothesis. Since nodes of the model do not have to correspond to real neurons, it makes representing new concepts much simpler by recruiting nodes from a pool of non-commissioned nodes. In learning, non-commissioned nodes are recruited to represent newly acquired concepts, and thus, they become commissioned. In addition, connections between nodes are modified to represent changes in the relationships between concepts. The firing of the commissioned nodes, innate and recruited, represents the presence of their concepts in the current event.

Memory records

When innately wired neurons fire, they represent the presence of their corresponding innate concepts. Although the individual innate concepts have been determined when the brain was created, the combinations in which they are activated depend on the particular experiences of the system. The brain can form and keep records of concepts that were present at the same time. It can also form and keep records of sequences of concepts that were present at different times. These records constitute the memory of the brain.

In principle, memory records can be formed by recruiting non-commissioned neurons to represent groups of firing neurons, and/or by modifying connections between commissioned neurons. How long such memory records last depends on how long the necessary connections between their neurons last. The brain has two major memory systems–short-term memory, and long-term memory. Their external manifestations are well documented, but their underlying processes still need to be fully understood. The model provides the basic tools–recruiting nodes and modifying ties–for representing both memory systems. How long ties last is a parameter of the model, which is left for the user to decide. The model can support a variety of mechanisms that reproduce the effects of short-term memory and long-term memory.

Connections

Part-whole and exemplar-class relationships

It has been observed that there is an order in the complexity of the concepts that are represented by cortical neurons. Neurons that are first to be activated by external stimuli represent concepts that are simpler than those represented by neurons that are activated afterwards. First, concepts that are represented by a small number of firing sensory neurons are represented. Then, various combinations of these secondary representations are grouped and represented by deeper cortical neurons, and so on. For example, neurons at the beginning of the signal-propagation-path in the visual cortex represent points and lines with different properties. Deeper neurons represent complex patterns, such as faces.

In neural networks, the propagation of signals from firing neurons to quiet ones may cause some of the latter to fire too. Since firing of neurons indicates that the concepts that they represent are present, the propagation of the activation implies that the presence of certain concepts induces the presence of other related ones. Because neurons in the cortex are organized according to the level of complexity of their concepts, it means that the presence of some simple concepts will elicit the presence of related complex concepts, and vice versa.

Humans can perceive the relationships between parts that make up a whole and the whole itself. **(In the following, the term 'item' may also be used to indicate a 'whole'.)** When all the parts are present, we can tell what is the whole. When we know that the whole is present, we can tell what are its parts. The relationship between a group of firing nodes and the firing node that represents them is similar to the relationship between the parts and their whole. Thus, neural-like circuitry can be used to model relationships between wholes and their parts, as illustrated in figure 1.2.

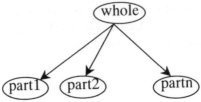

Figure 1.2:   A connectionist drawing of parts-whole relationships between nodes.

An arrow with a thick head represents a bi-directional connection. An arrow like those in figure 1.2 indicates a whole-part relationship. The direction of the arrow indicates that the presence of the whole implies the presence of each and every one of its parts, and the presence of all the parts implies the presence of the whole. The presence of any part by itself does not imply the presence of the whole. Invoking the parts when the whole is invoked can be done in one step or gradually. Most often, when a whole is invoked, only some of its pertinent parts are invoked. The brain can invoke more parts if it is requested to do so.

It is generally accepted that in real neurons information can propagate only in one direction. Based on that, if information propagates from neurons that represent parts to neurons that represent their whole, it cannot propagate back using the same physical pathways. On the other hand, many areas of the brain have reciprocal connections between them. Through such indirect connections, a firing neuron can send feedback signals and affect neurons that caused it to fire. It is acceptable for connectionist models to rely on architecture and mechanisms that do not have exact counterparts in biological neural networks. The bi-directional connections that are used in this connectionist model replicate only the functionality of information flow between neurons, and not its detailed supporting anatomy and physiology.

In addition to whole-part relationships, humans can perceive also class-exemplar relationships. We can tell if any member of a given group of objects belongs to a given class. If we know the class, we can list its members. For example, we can classify A, **a**, and *a* as exemplars of the letter 'a'. When asked to write the letter A, we can do it in various fonts. This class-exemplar relationship can be modeled by arrows that connect nodes that represent the exemplars and a node that represents the class. Figure 1.3 illustrates exemplar-class relationships between nodes:

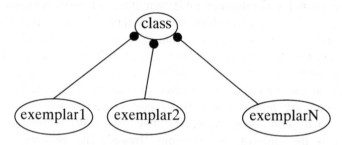

Figure 1.3: A connectionist model of exemplars-class relationships

The circular headed arrows represent exemplar-class relationship. Whenever any one of the exemplars is present, the presence of its class is implied. When a class is present, the presence of any of its exemplars is not implied automatically. The exemplar-class relationship is represented by a bi-directional connection between the respective nodes. Like the part-whole relationship, the connectionist network that represents exemplar-class relationships replicates the functionality of biological networks and not their actual anatomy and physiology.

A whole-node expresses the concept that when all its parts are present, it is present too, and when the whole-node is present, its part are present too. If $p_1, p_2, ..., p_n$ represent the n parts of the whole-node W, the parts-whole relationship, as expressed by the synaptic weight, represents the logical statements:

if $(p_1$ AND p_2 AND, ..., $p_n)$ then W

and

if (W) then $(p_1$ AND p_2 AND, ..., $p_n)$ [1.2]

Similarly, when an exemplar-node is present, its class-node C is present, and when C is present, any of its m exemplars $e_1, e_2, ..., e_m$ may be present:

if $(e_1$ OR e_2 OR, ..., $e_m)$ then C

and

$$[1.3]$$

$$\text{if (C) then } (e_1 \text{ OR } e_2 \text{ OR, ..., } e_m)$$

In artificial intelligence (AI), semantic networks represent information entities and the relationships between them. The information entities are represented by nodes and the relationships by arcs. All kinds of arcs have been used in AI. Any relationship may have its own arc. The approach here is that only two basic relationships are represented by arcs. All the other relationships, which are represented in some AI semantic networks by their own arcs, are represented here by nodes and the two basic relationships: whole-part and class-exemplar. The two-way whole-part relationship contains the one-way relationship '**has-a**'; the two-way exemplar-class relationship contains the one-way '**is-a**' relationship, which are widely used in AI. A given node in a semantic network can play different roles. It can be a part, a whole, an exemplar, and a class at the same time. These properties depend not on the node itself, but how it relates to other nodes.

A group of activated nodes represents the presence of a **scene**. Some of the nodes that make up a scene may be activated by external factors. Due to the connections between the nodes, externally activated nodes may cause the activation of other nodes, thus adding them to the scene. The presence of some information entities in a scene is thus inferred from the presence of others. Here are some examples: (1) An externally activated whole node may activate its part nodes. (2) When all the parts of whole are externally activated, their whole node is also activated and becomes a part of the scene. (3) When an exemplar node is externally activated, its class node is also activated.

New nodes may be added to a semantic network, as it acquires new information. For example, class nodes may add new exemplar nodes, and exemplars may be added to newly defined class nodes. Nodes may also be deleted from a semantic network. That occurs, for example, when noise has been included as part of a whole, and new experiences indicate that it should be trimmed out.

An information entity can become an exemplar of a class in three ways. *First*, arbitrarily. For example, inanimate nouns in some languages belong to one of two gender classes. These affiliations are arbitrary, and they may vary from one language to another. *Second*, by a common part. For example, the class of green objects. Each member has the color green. *Third*, by a common association. For example, flute and violin are musical instruments. Class affiliation due to a common association is a generalization of the idea of class affiliation due to a common part. In both cases, the affiliation of the exemplar to the class is determined by an association with a third entity, or a **pointer**. In simple cases, the pointer is a part of the exemplar. In more general cases, the pointer is associated with the exemplar in a prescribed way. These differences are illustrated in figure 1.4.

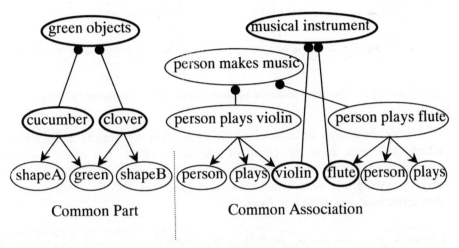

Common Part   Common Association

Figure 1.4: Example circuitry for class affiliation bases upon common part and upon common association.

Pointers

Wholes may become exemplars of a class based on some common features that they share. A set of features that characterizes a whole as an exemplar of a class will be called here a **pointer** of that **class**. The features that constitute a pointer may be represented by their own node. This pointer node will be in between the nodes that represent its features and the node that represents its class. Similarly, a set of parts that are characteristic to one whole will be called here a **pointer** of that **whole**. A pointer of a whole identifies that whole when some of its parts are invoked.

Pointers embody fundamental generalization rules of the system. They enable the identification of wholes when only some of their parts are invoked, and the assignment of new wholes as exemplars to given classes. A pointer represents a cluster of parts, which is specific to one class or to one whole.

Different arrows can be used in drawings of networks to indicate the various semantic relationships between information entities, which are represented by nodes. The arrows do not display the synaptic weights of the involved connections. The basic semantic relationships are illustrated in figure 1.5:

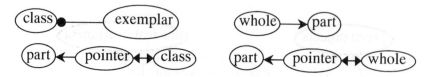

Figure 1.5: The basic semantic relationships between information entities.

Nodes may also be connected to each other by simple connections, which determine how the firing of one node affects the other, without providing any additional information about other associated nodes or the reverse association. Such connections and processes will be represented by thin arrowheads, as shown in figure 1.6

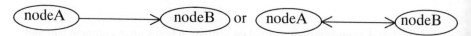

Figure 1.6: Notations for simple connections between nodes.

The single arrow indicates that firing of nodeA causes the firing of nodeB. The bi-directional arrow indicates that whenever one node fires, the other also fires. That makes the two nodes identical from the network's point of view.

An inhibitory connection from nodeA to nodeB will be denoted by a squared arrowhead:

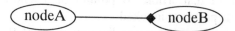

Figure 1.7: Notation for inhibitory connection.

Negation is not a transitive relationship. If A is not a part of B, and B is not a part of C it does not mean that A is not a part of C.

The entire set of associations that a node has can be represented by four bundles of bi-directional synaptic connections, as shown in figure 1.8:

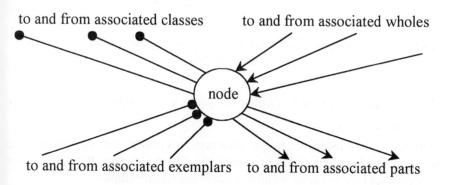

Figure 1.8: The four semantic bundles of a node.

Explicit and implicit representations, inheritance

Since the whole-part and class-exemplar relationships are transitive (e.g. if A is a part of B and B is a part of C then A is also a part of C), only **contiguous** associations will be explicitly recorded by the model. For example, A is a part of B will be explicitly recorded, and B is a part of C will be explicitly recorded, while A is a part of C will not be explicitly recorded. Being a part of C is a property that A inherits from B.

Classes may have their own parts. These parts are properties that all the exemplars of the class inherit, even if these properties are not defining parts of the exemplars. For example, 'mortal' is a part of the class 'live animals'. It may not be a defining part of any live animal, as perceived by the brain based upon its sensory inputs, but all live animals have this property. In general, part-whole relationships, when not recorded explicitly by a connection between the whole-node and the part-node, can be recorded implicitly. The whole is an explicit exemplar of the class, and the part is an explicit part of the class, as figure 1.9 shows:

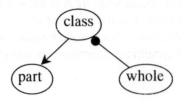

Figure 1.9: implicit part-whole relationship (e.g. whole=human; class=live animal; part=mortal).

Representing whole-part, class-exemplar, and pointer relationships by synaptic weights

Semantic relationships between information entities can be modeled as relationships between nodes in a network. The nodes play the roles of the concepts, and the synaptic weights encode the relationships.

The following expressions detail how semantic relationships between information entities can be represented by synaptic weights in a network. The notations are according to [1.1].

If node j represents the whole and nodes i are its contiguous parts, then $\sum_i \sigma_{ij} \geq 1$

If node i represents the whole and node j represents any one of its contiguous parts then $\sigma_{ij} \geq 1$.   [1.4]

If node i represent the class and node j represents any one of its contiguous exemplars then $\sigma_{ij} \geq 1$

If node j, whose parts are nodes i, is a pointer to node m then: $\sum_i \sigma_{ij} \geq 1$, and $\sigma_{ji} \geq 1$, and $\sigma_{jm} \geq 1$.

Other connections between nodes

When asked to name a class whose exemplar is 'dog' we know to come up with 'animal', or another valid answer. When asked to name as exemplar of 'animal' we may answer 'dog', or 'cat', or some other appropriate answer

We do not know what brain circuitry is involved in providing such answers, but there is no doubt that these are processes that the brain performs routinely. Each of the four semantic relationships that may exist between two nodes, namely: part-whole, exemplar-class, and their inverses, are represented in the model by two links of opposite polarities and synaptic weights according to [1.4]. This is done to facilitate information handling by the model. It does not imply that such connections really exist between neurons.

In addition to these connections, two nodes may be connected by one-directional links, such as halves of expressions [1.2] or [1.3]. When only the first half of [1.2] is represented by a link, (i.e. when only "if (p_1 AND p_2 AND, ..., p_n) then W" is represented) the presence of the parts would activate the node that represents the whole. However, if the whole has been activated through a mechanism that did not involve its parts, signals would not be able to propagate to the part-nodes and to activate them. Situations like this occur in the brain. For example, the perception of the color of a point is created by signals from three light sensors, which sense the point. These three sensors may be considered part-nodes of the node that represents of the point's perceived color. When they are quiet, it is impossible to activate those part-nodes by propagating signals from the firing whole-node that represents the perceived color. We cannot tell what fundamental colors have contributed to the perceived color. One-directional links are indicated in diagrams by arrows with thin heads. They may have any synaptic weight.

2.   COMPUTERS, AI, AND THE MODEL

Computers in general

The following is a general description of some common principles on which most computers operate. Different computers may use variations of these principles, or may use some other principles altogether. The purpose of describing these principles here is to help us focus on some fundamental issues in the function of computers, and to compare and contrast them with similar issues that are relevant to the brain.

Computers are devices that manipulate symbols. The symbols that we key into a computer consist of letters, numbers, and other special characters. In the computer, these symbols are encoded as binary words, so that the computer can handle them. The computer manipulates this information, and its output consists of various combinations of these symbols. The computer sends these symbols to a variety of devices that, in turn, interpret them and generate the output in its final form, such as text on the monitor's screen.

A basic computer consists of a central processing unit (CPU) and peripheral units, which are connected to the CPU. Typical peripheral units are main memory, disk drives, terminal, and printer. The entire computer's operation is synchronized by an internal clock. The clock sends time-tick signals that trigger and coordinate the activities of the various units of the computer.

A CPU has three main parts: control unit, arithmetic-logic unit (ALU), and registers. The control unit controls the operations of the ALU on the data, which is temporarily stored in the registers. Data registers are used to store the data processed by the CPU. For example, if we want to add the numbers 3 and 5, they have to be placed in binary form in designated registers. The CPU gets also the binary code for the operation 'add'. The control unit activates a circuitry that adds the two numbers and places the result 8 in a designated register. In addition to data, designated registers store

17

instructions that are sent to and from the peripherals. Port registers store data and instruction that are communicated to and from the peripherals. For example, if the number 17 has to be copied to memory cell 512, these numbers and the code for moving a number into memory location are stored at designated registers. The control unit activates the appropriate circuitry, so that the transfer is executed. Flag registers store information about the last operation of the CPU. For example, consider the operation of adding to the number in register A to the number in register B, and keeping the answer in register A. It may happen that register A is too small to store the sum, even if each of the two added numbers were valid (there was an overflow). The user needs to know that the final number in register A is not the required outcome, even though it may look like a legitimate binary word. The flag register will provide this important information.

An executed CPU instruction modifies the data stored in its registers. These data are considered the variables of the instruction. Different instructions may depend on different number of variables. Some instructions do not depend on any variable. For example: "store the number 0 in register A".

The CPU operates in cycles that can be divided into several steps. First, an instruction is brought to the instruction register. A pointer is then set to point to the next instruction. The type of the residing instruction is then interpreted. If the instruction calls for data from the memory, the data is fetched to the designated registers. Now the instruction is executed, and the results are stored in their proper place. That terminates the instruction cycle, and a new cycle begins. These steps may happen sequentially or they may overlap in time. An idling computer executes cycles that continuously scan designated registers for a new instruction to be executed. The details of the circuitries that carry out an instruction are transparent to the programmer. Designing them has been the responsibility of the creators of the computer.

The memory consists of cells that store information as binary words. (A word consists of bytes, and each byte consists of eight bits). The number of bits in a memory word (the size of the word) may change from computer to computer. Each memory cell has an address. The address of a memory cell is also encoded as a binary word, whose size may vary from computer to computer, and may be different from the size of the data words. At any given time, a memory cell has one address that the CPU can use, and each valid address used by the CPU points to one memory cell.

The communication between the CPU and the memory is routed through the CPU's memory-port-register. The CPU accesses the information stored in a memory cell by specifying the address of the cell, and the code of the operation to be executed on the data. Some of the possible operations on the data are: read (copy the contents of the cell to a CPU's register), write (copy the contents of a CPU's register to the memory cell), or reset. The CPU can calculate the numerical values of pointers to memory cells, as well as the contents of memory cells. By manipulating pointers, the CPU controls where information is stored, or from where it is retrieved. By manipulating the contents of cells, the CPU affects the stored information itself.

The memory can store programs, which are sequences of instructions to the CPU. When the CPU executes a program, it copies one instruction at a time into the instruction register, and executes it. The CPU then copies the next instruction, executes it, and so on, until the end of the program. At that time, the computer returns to idling mode, ready for a new instruction or a new program.

A machine language program is a sequence of CPU instructions. A high level program is a set of instructions, each of which represents a group of CPU instructions. Computers have programs that translate high level programs into machine language programs. The high level programs are first compiled and then linked with other compiled programs, as necessary, to form the executable machine language programs, which are used by the CPU in run time.

Data representation in computers and brain models

The primary duty of the brain is to enable the body to function in its environment. The brain gets encoded information about the body and the environment, processes it based on its innate wiring and its learned information, and issues encoded response instructions to the pertinent parts of the body. The brain can access its stored data, manipulate it, and store the results of such manipulations. The data that the brain stores contains records of various stimuli that the brain received and the operation that the brain performed.

Feature detectors

The periphery of the nervous system consists of sensory neurons and motor neurons, which are represented by binary nodes in the model. Each peripheral node can be viewed as representing an information bit in a huge binary array, which represents events that occur outside of the system. A firing peripheral node is represented in this peripheral array as a bit of one, and an un-stimulated node as a bit of zero.

Activated peripheral nodes cause the activation of inner nodes. In this sense, these inner nodes represent the peripheral patterns by which they have been activated. If the connections between the peripheral nodes and these inner nodes are innate, the inner nodes act as innate feature detectors. Whenever a feature (a pattern of firing nodes) occurs in the periphery, its feature detector node detects it, and fires. On the other hand, if these connections are learned, the inner nodes act as an acquired feature detector. An acquired feature detector represents fragments of events that have happened in the periphery. These memories are re-invoked whenever their corresponding patterns recur in the outside world.

As information keeps propagating further inside, some activated nodes will represent peripheral patterns combined with representations of the brain's own operations. Again, if the channels leading to these internal nodes are not innate, these nodes reflect the recurrence of past experiences.

Memory addresses and contents

There are some similarities between invoking memories in the model and accessing memory cells in computers. In computers, the addresses of a memory cells are expressed by relatively short binary words that have a fixed number of bits. The address of a given cell is encoded as a specific combination of bits of one and bits of zero in the address word. For example, words of twenty bits provide more than million different addresses. In the model, the peripheral nodes may be regarded as a huge binary array, or a word. A group of peripheral nodes that fire may cause a cascade of intermediate firing nodes that ends in a single firing node. This final node is representing the initial group of the firing peripheral nodes. Since the firing peripheral nodes can be viewed as bits of one in their array, it can be said that these firing peripheral nodes express the address of that final firing node, which also represents them.

There are, however, few differences between addressing memories by computers and by the model.

- In computers, the values of all the bits in the address-word have to be specified in order to access the memory cell. In the model, only a small part of the huge peripheral array participates in invoking a representing node.
- In computers, each memory cell has one address, while in the model, one node may be a representation of various peripheral patterns.
- In computers, a valid address corresponds to one memory cell, while in the model a pattern of peripheral active nodes (an address) may invoke several representing nodes.
- Computers and the model may accept addresses that do not correspond to any memory location. In computers, this is referred to as 'address outside the range'. In the model, this happens when a novel peripheral pattern, which is not represented by a real or virtual node, occurs.
- In computers, a CPU can access a memory cell only if its address is specified, while in the model it is possible to access nodes by specifying their relationships to other nodes that do not belong to the peripheral array.

In computers, the meaning of the content of a memory cell is provided by the programmer. In the brain and in the model, the meaning of the content of an internal node is determined by its relationships with other nodes. The address of a node is a part of its meaning. It represents a group of co-active peripheral nodes. The relationship between peripheral address nodes and their representing node is parts-to-whole. A node will usually have various relationships with other nodes. These relationships can be of any type: part-whole, whole-part, exemplar-class, and class-exemplar. The ensemble of all these relationships is the information content of a memory node.

Operations in computers and in the model

Operations and operation units

An operation in a CPU, such as adding two numbers, uses designated input and output registers. First, the variables are copied into the input registers of the operation. Then, a computation unit, which consists of an appropriate electronic circuitry, gets a start signal and does the actual computation. Finally, the result is placed in the output registers of the operation. The result may be a number that has a certain meaning for the user or a coded instructions to other parts of the computer, such as to store a number at a certain memory cell. The electronic operations that were employed by the computation unit to reach its results are transparent to the user that writes the program.

Similarly, the mechanics of some of the operation of the model would be transparent to its users. These operations would be executed by special operation units that operate in coordination with the regular nodes of the model, and that affect the state of the nodes. For example, an operation unit may establish new synapses between firing nodes of the model. In practice, the operation unit would get signals from regular nodes, and then summon the simulation program to establish the new synapses, in accordance with these signals. Biological systems have inherent special mechanisms to modify synaptic strengths between neurons. The details of such activities are beyond the scope of the model. Moreover, the model should function properly with different operation units that perform the same task. Operation units are handled by the simulation program that executes their requests.

An operation unit contains three main sub-units: (1) Input slots–designated nodes to which the nodes that represent the actual input are temporarily connected. (2) Output slots–designated nodes to which nodes that represent the output of the operation are temporarily connected. (3) An operator sub unit–a circuitry through which the input signals flow and which creates the output, according to the given input. The output may be a pattern of firing nodes, or a call to the simulation program. Like the input slots and the output slots, the operators themselves are also concepts of the system. As such, each operator is represented by a node. This node, which will be called op-rep, fires whenever the operator is active, thus representing its presence to the rest of the system. Figure 2.1 illustrates the nodes and sub-units that make-up an operation unit.

An operation may have two kinds of outcome. First, a node or a group of nodes may be activated. Second, changes may be made in the circuitry of the network. These changes include modifications of existing ties and creations of new ties between existing and recruited nodes. For example, edge detection is an operation that is performed by the brain. In the model, edge detection may be done by an edge detection unit. When an active pattern of nodes that contain an edge is connected to the input slots of that unit, it will detect the edge, using procedures that are transparent to the user. The unit would identify the nodes that form the edge, recruit whole-node to represent that edge, and connect the identified nodes as part-nodes to the recruited node that represents the edge. The recruited edge-node would then be connected to the output slot of the unit. In addition, the detection unit may fire one of its dedicated nodes, to signal that an edge has been detected.

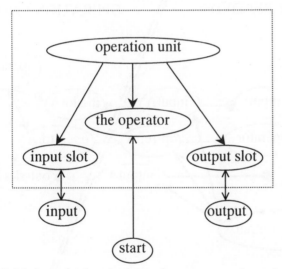

Figure 2.1: Nodes and sub-units that make-up an operation unit (inside dashed box), and outside nodes that are involved in an operation.

The model's equivalent of a computer's program is a chain of operation units. An activated output node of one active operation unit becomes the activated input of the next operation unit, and so on. The model has a 'start' node, that activates the first operation in the program, and an 'end' node, which is activated when the program finishes its last operation. In the model, different programs may execute simultaneously (parallel processing).

Records of operations

In addition to executing operations, the system is able to create and keep memory-records describing the details of its operations. These records are organized such that they could be retrieved systematically. Figure 2.2 illustrates how a record of a certain operation that took place (operationA), and consisted of certain input (inputA) and certain output (outputA) is recorded by the network.

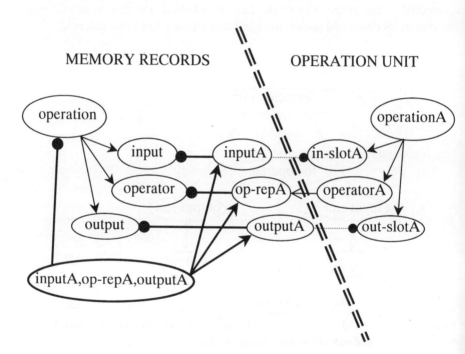

Figure 2.2: Creating a memory record of an operation: A certain inputA served as an input to a certain operationA, and a certain outputA resulted (right side of the figure). The general concept of an operation and its parts are also represented by nodes (denoted as 'operation', 'input', 'operator', and 'output' in the left side of the figure). To record the current event, memory-nodes inputA, op-repA, and outputA, recruit an item node to represent them, and form new connections with nodes that

represent memory concepts (heavy lines in the figure). They become parts of a node that is recruited to represent the memory of the entire event (inputA,op_repA,outputA). Exemplar-class connections are also established between the nodes that represent the current event and the permanent concept nodes (left side of figue), so that the roles of the current nodes in the event are also recorded. For example, the node 'inputA' is part of the memory record 'inputA,op_repA,outputA', which is a record of the entire event. 'InputA' becomes also an exemplar of the memory concept 'input', thus encoding the role of 'inputA' in the record 'inputA,op_repA,outputA'.

A general operation is a threesome relationship between a list of input variables, the operator itself, and a list of outcome variables. An operation can be in an **assertive** mode or in **probative** mode. In the assertive mode, nodes that represent the outcome are invoked as a result of the actual operation of the operator on the input nodes. The right side of figure 2.2 shows the nodes that are involved in an assertive operation. The left-hand side of figure 2.2 shows the nodes that are involved in probative operations. In probative operations, an outcome is invoked without the activation of the operator itself. This is, basically, a retrieval from the memory. When a probative operation is performed, part of the threesome–the given–is provided, and another part–the unknown–has to be retrieved.

In formal notations, an operation can be written as (input,operator,outcome). A question mark will signify the unknown. An assertive operation will be written as (input,operator,?). A number of probative operations can be performed on a memory recored of an operation. For example, the retrieval request (input,operator,outcome?) activates the outcome node of a memory-record, if the input node and the operator node are specified. This is done entirely in the circuitry of the left side of figure 2.2. There are several retrieval requests for any given memory record of an operation, e.g. (input?,operator,outcome) or (input,operator?,outcome). In addition to these retrieval requests, the memory can also be probed for the existence of an entire record: ?(input,operator,outcom)?. The answer to such a probe is yes or no, which is provided by a dedicated node in the circuitry of the probative operation.

In some situations, computers keep a log of the operations that they have performed. The brain does it as a matter of routine, and relies on such 'logs', in its future activities.

Accessing data and outcome flags

An information entity in a computer's memory has to be copied to a register of the CPU in order to participate in a computation. Accessing information in the memory and copying it are parts of a basic operation that the CPU does. If the address used by the CPU is legitimate, i.e. belongs to one of the memory's cells, the data in this cell will be copied to a CPU's register, and the CPU would be able to proceed with the computation. The address of the memory cell has to explicitly reside in the CPU before its contents can be copied. Sometimes, addresses are given implicitly; e.g., the contents of register A plus one. In such cases, the CPU has to calculate an explicit address, place it in the data-address-register, and only then access the data.

In the model, in order to explicitly participate in a computation, an information entity has to be invoked, i.e. its representing node has to fire. One way of invoking a node that represents a whole is to invoke all its parts. For example, the basic visual features of a familiar face that we look at activate a node that represents that face. This is the model's analog of the CPU accessing data based on its explicit address. However, a number of situations that occur in the brain and in the model do not have a CPU counterpart.

- A group of firing nodes may activate one node that represents only some of them. For example, when we hear a sentence that contains an unfamiliar word, the familiar words invoke their representation, but no representation is invoked by the unfamiliar word, because it is not yet represented in the brain.

- A group of firing nodes may activate a number of nodes that, as a group, represent the entire original group, but there is no one node that represents the entire event. For example, a person that we know puts on a new hat. The person and the hat each have representing nodes, but the person wearing the hat is not yet represented by a node.

- A group of firing nodes may activate a number of nodes that represent only some of the original nodes. This is a combination of the previous cases.

- A group of firing nodes may not activate any node at all. This happens when the event is new.

To make the information about the type of the invoked outcome available to the rest of the system, the brain should have something similar to a CPU's flag register, which provides meta-information about the quality of invoked information. Indeed, it seems that the brain has mechanisms to that effect.

We are aware when any of those situations occurs. We can tell which parts of a given scene invoked their representation, and which part, if any, remains un-represented. This is true when not only parts have to invoke their representing whole-node, but also when the brain has to retrieve information based on general specifications.

The basic operations and instructions of the model

Basic operation and structure of nodes

Every higher level programming language, such as Pascal or C++, has a set of basic instructions with which all its programs are composed. For an instruction to be executed, it has first to be translated into a 'machine language' code, which consists of more fundamental instructions that interact directly with the hardware. Even a machine level instruction initiates operation of many fundamental electronic circuits in the CPU. Overall, a lot of transparent activity takes place between the original higher level instruction and its final outcome. Similarly, propagation of signals between neurons can be viewed as a 'machine level' operation of the brain. Understanding the operation of the brain would be facilitated by the understanding the 'higher level languages' that the brain may be using. The model presented here proposes such a language, which can be used to program all its own activities. In addition to regulating signals that propagate from node to node in the network, similarly to signals that propagate in a network of standard neurons (figure 1.1), the language has also instructions that describe higher level processes. The nodes of the model have hardware components that accommodate those higher level instructions. These components do not represent parts of real neurons. Rather, they represent processes that the brain can perform on its neurons. Macroscopically, there are indications that the brain performs these processes. In many cases, it is not known how the neuronal circuitry is involved in these operations. These features of the nodes of the model are discussed next.

The data channels of a node are divided into four main bundles, according to the roles that the node can play with respect to other nodes. The bundles are parts-to-whole (where whole, or item, is the role of the node), exemplars to class (the node is the class), wholes to part (the node is the part), and exemplar-to classes (the node is the exemplar). Each bundle contains bi-directional connections between the node and other nodes. The synaptic weights of the ties encode the relationships between the nodes, as detailed in [1.4]. Being able to use this encoded information and to manipulate it is essential for the model. The model has several sets of basic operations that are used for that purpose. This is the model's analog of a CPU's basic operations such as addition, multiplication, logical operations, etc. The first set of basic operations are the basic invoking instructions. They invoke an outcome based on its association with the given input. These are:

- Invoke X whose part is A.
- Invoke X whose whole is A.
- Invoke X whose class is A.
- Invoke X whose exemplar is A.

The letter A stands for a single node, and X stands for a list of nodes. Formally, these operations can be written as

- (A, invoke whole, X).
- (A, invoke part, X).
- (A, invoke exemplar, X).
- (A, invoke class, X).

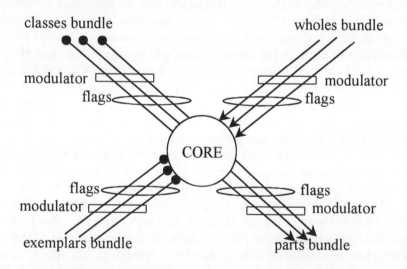

Figure 2.3: A node and its bundles, modulators, and flags.

A signal from a firing node reaches all it bundles. In order to be able to carry out a basic invoking instruction, it is necessary to be able to block on demand the irrelevant bundles. That will ensure that the outgoing signals will propagate only via the desired bundle. Once the signals have entered the target nodes, they may invoke too many or too few nodes. For having the situation under control, each bundle has two "hardware elements": a modulator and flags. The modulators are controlled from outside by bundle-control nodes. The modulators do not affect incoming signals. A modulator can completely block outgoing signals in its bundle, or modulate their intensity. The flags fire when a target node, which is stimulated through the bundle, fires, thus providing information on the efficacy of the invoking instruction. These functional parts of a node are illustrated in figure 2.3.

The processes of executing these four basic invoking operations are similar. They are based on activating the given node after disabling all its unneeded bundles. For example, in the execution of: 'invoke X whose part is A', all the bundles of node A are disabled, except the part-to-wholes bundle. Then, node A is activated, and it sends signals to all its whole nodes. The disabling is carried out by the modulation units. Each outgoing bundle has its modulation unit. A modulation unit controls the efficacy of the signals that flow through the bundle. It can completely inhibit signals propagation through the bundle, or it can multiply their intensities by a controllable **modulation-factor** m, where $m \geq 0$. In the example, the value of m at the 'to wholes' bundle is set to a very small value. Then, it is continuously increased until a whole of A is invoked. At this time, the flag of the 'to wholes' bundle fires, indicating that one whole has been invoked. The execution of 'invoke X whose part is A' is then complete. If the modulation reaches its maximum value without invoking any whole, the execution terminates at that. By increasing or decreasing the value of m, the number of invoked entities can be controlled. The modulators and the flags interact only with information that flows out of the node.

A modulation operation can be directed to a single node, or broadcast to a group of nodes. Modulation is a basic element of scanning operations. In scanning, different exemplars of a class are invoked one at a time, and become available to other computations.

Not all the nodes in the system have all the sub-structures illustrated in figure 2.3. The absence of a sub-structure will mean that the node cannot execute the particular function that the sub-structure supports. For example, a node having only the incoming ties of the parts bundle will be activated by its parts but will not be able to directly activate them.

Recruiting nodes and ties

There are two kinds of nodes in the system: commissioned and non-commissioned (or free). Commissioned nodes have associations with other nodes, while free nodes do not have association with any other node. A free node becomes commissioned when it becomes associated with another node. A commissioned node becomes free when all its associations with other nodes are cancelled.

There are four basic recruiting operations. They recruit a free node X, and assign to it a specified relationship to a given node A. Similar to the basic invoking operations, these are:

- (A, recruit whole, X).
- (A, recruit part, X).
- (A, recruit exemplar, X).
- (A, recruit class, X).

There are four basic association operations, which have corresponding instructions. They form new associations between nodes A and B, which are already commissioned:

- (A, make whole of, B).
- (A, make part of, B).
- (A, make exemplar of, B).
- (A, make class of B).

Each of these operations has its reverse, in which an established association is dissociated. A node that loses all its associations becomes free.

It was mentioned earlier that due to the transitivity of the class-exemplar and whole-part relationships, only contiguous associations are physically recorded by the network. Normally, only contiguous classes of the exemplar, or contiguous parts of the whole will be invoked as a result of the basic invoking operations. In order to invoke non-contiguous associations, the instruction **explicate** is appended, once or several times, to the basic invoking operation. The invoked non-contiguous nodes may be physically connected to the exemplar or to the whole by basic association operations.

These connections may be eliminated by the basic dissociation operations, as needed.

Real-time and instruction-time

It takes time for the CPU to execute its various operations. Different instructions may require different times to be completed. An internal clock provides time ticks by which the CPU coordinates the operations of various circuitries that are involved in the execution of an instruction. From the perspective of an outsider, the relevant state of the computer, i.e. the contents of its registers and memory cells, is available at discrete time intervals. The CPU does its computations between those intervals. In the brain, events are represented by firing neurons. It takes time for signals to propagate from one neuron to another and to cause neurons to fire. This is similar to the time interval that the CPU needs to execute an operation. In the model, the state of the system at a given time is determined by the firing nodes at that particular time. Time is divided into intervals, which represent real time. The simulation program figures out everything that happens within a time interval, and updates the state of the involved nodes at the end of that time interval.

The brain probably does not rely on a central clock to precisely pre-determine the execution time of each operation. It probably senses that the outcome of an operation is available, and moves on to the next operation. This approach is used also by the model.

Labeling

The brain carries out many operations at the same time. It is not known if and how the brain groups its firing neurons according to the operations that occur at the same time. It is possible that some resonance or reverberations characterize all the nodes that belong to such a group. It is also possible that some 'token', which is passed from node to node as activation propagates in the network, is used for such identification. One of the features of the model is parallel processing, meaning that different operations may take place at the same time. Concepts that participate in an operation are present in the system, and therefore they are represented by firing nodes. A node may be accessible to several operation units, and therefore firing nodes need to be identified according to the operation in which they participate. The model provides for temporary labeling of nodes by their controlling operation units.

These labels, which can be realized by temporal activation patterns that are superimposed on the activation of the nodes, can be used to restrict the interaction between nodes only to those nodes that carry the same label. A node that participates in several operations at the same time will carry the labels of all of those operations.

Organization of the model

The flow of information to and from the peripheral arrays and the processing of the information are performed in modules. This is pretty much what happens in the brain. In the model, each of the five basic senses, the motor system, and the feeling system has its own module. There are also various association modules, in which information from different modules is merged. The modules consist of compartments that process data and relay information to other compartments. The compartments have input arrays, output arrays, and intermediary processing and storage units. The compartments of all the peripheral modules and some association modules have special structures for processing information, called **arenas**.

The arenas

An arena in the brain is similar to a TV screen. A TV screen has a matrix of pixels. Moving images are displayed on the screen by activating the appropriate pixels at the appropriate time. Similarly, a matrix of nodes represents the field of view in the visual module. Another matrix represents points on the body's surface in the somatosensory module, and so on. A sequence of events in the visual field may thus be represented as a sequence of activated patterns of nodes in the visual arena. A pixel of a color TV is a cluster consisting of red, green and blue dots. Similarly, a point in the visual field is represented by a cluster of nodes (**pixel's-cluster**) in the visual arena. Each of these nodes represents a different feature of the visual point, such as color, brightness, direction of motion (if the pixel is a part of a moving image), being at the edge, etc. Any active node in a pixel-cluster represents the presence of its feature in that pixel of the field of view. Similarly, nodes in the pixel-clusters of the somatosensory arena will represent pressure, temperature, pain, wetness, etc. of that particular body pixel. Pixel-cluster nodes may be activated directly by peripheral nodes, or by intermediary nodes of the same or other modules.

When pixel-clusters of the peripheral modules are activated by outside factors, they represent real external events. Pixel-clusters may also be activated by internal nodes. In such cases, they represent simulations of external events, or thoughts about external events, or mental pictures. For example, real two cars moving head on into each other are represented in the visual arena as two moving patterns of firing nodes. This is initiated by light stimuli to peripheral sensory nodes. The statement 'two cars moving head on into each other', which originates at another module, invokes some parts of those moving patterns in the visual arena. This is a simulation of the representation of the real event.

Detectors and projectors

The pixel-clusters are connected to circuits of nodes, which will be called detectors. These detectors analyze the features in the events that are displayed in their arena. The detectors forward their findings to other nodes in the same or in other modules. To continue the previous example, the detectors in the visual module, which simulates the two cars, will detect a simulated collision, and forward this information to other units. Each arena has a large number of detectors, which process simultaneously the data displayed in it.

In many situations, detectors operate as classifiers. Their firing indicates that a given whole belongs to their specific class. Figure 2.4 illustrates the phases of a classification process. An information structure, consisting of a whole node and its parts, is active. The nodes of the structure are connected to the detector, and activate its inner circuitry. The detector detects that the information structure possesses critical features, which make the whole eligible to belong to the class that it detects. The detector activates the class node of the class. If the whole is not yet an exemplar of that class, a tie is formed between the whole node and the class node to record this finding.

In the previous example, whole becomes an exemplar of a class because parts that belong to the whole satisfy the qualifying requirements. A detector that analyzed these parts initiates the formation of the exemplar-to-class connection between the whole and the class-node. However, as mentioned earlier, there are instances when wholes are eligible to become exemplars of a class not because of their internal properties but due to their relation to an

external event. In such cases, the detection and the classification are
performed by units that are more complex.

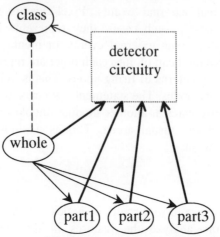

Figure 2.4: Schematics of a classifier.

Each arena has also its specialized projectors. Projectors activate patterns
of nodes in the arena, in a way that simulates the essentials of real events.
For example, the word 'siren' activates a projector in the auditory arena that
simulates the sound of a siren. This projector consists of fundamental
projectors, which activate representations of basic sounds in the typical
sequence of a siren. Projected patterns can be analyzed in conjunction with
representations of real events by the detectors of the arena. The detectors of
an arena can process real information, that originates at the input of the
arena, as well as simulated information. The results of such analysis become
available to the rest of the system. For example, before crossing the street,
we look at the traffic. The real images of the moving cars, together with
projections of our would-be-position with respect to them should we cross
the street, are analyzed by the detectors of the visual arena. The outcome is
forwarded to other parts of the system, where decisions are made. Each
arena contains many detectors and projectors, which may operate at the same
time. These operators are triggered by sets of active nodes, constituting their
inputs. The outputs of the operations are other sets of active nodes and new
pieces of circuitry, which are added to the existing ones. When a number of
operators operate in parallel, it may be important to relate the output of an

operation to its input, and not to mistakenly attribute it to the input of a different operator. For example, if car A is moving to the right and, at the same time, car B is moving to the left, the detected properties 'moving to the right' and 'moving to the left' have to be assigned to the appropriate cars. By using labels, each operator can identify its own input and output, and relate to them properly, as needed.

In addition to detectors and projectors, each arena provides information to memory nodes, where records of representations of events that involved its detectors and projectors are stored.

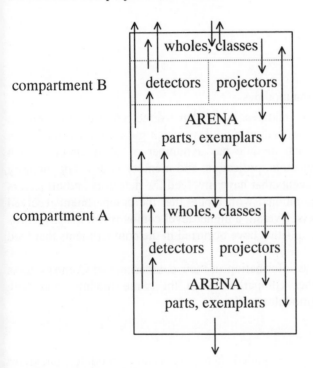

Figure 2.5: Paths of information flow between the elements of two compartments.

The compartments

A compartment consists of an arena and its support circuitries (figure 2.5). The pixel nodes of the arena represent parts and exemplars, which are handled by the compartment. The detectors of the compartment analyze the patterns of activated pixels, and cause the activation of the compartment's whole and class nodes. Activated pixels, detectors, whole, and class nodes can relay their signals to other compartments. Whole and class nodes can activate projector nodes, which activate patterns of pixels in the arena. A compartment receives its input through the input pixels, and through whole and class nodes. Both kinds of nodes–those representing reality and those representing memories–are found in a compartment. The detectors and the projectors are the operation units within a compartment. Real events are recorded and their memories are retrieved as explained above. Figure 2.5 illustrates the various paths of information flows that may exist between two compartments.

The modules

Peripheral and association modules

In addition to peripheral modules, which have direct connections with the outside, there are also association modules, which get all their information from other modules. Each module has a number of compartments, each containing an arena, detectors, projectors, and memory nodes. The memory nodes keep records of events that have involved the detectors and projectors of that compartment, combined with inputs that the compartment received from other compartments. Overall, a higher level compartment keeps records of conjunctions of concepts that have occurred in the compartments that feed it.

The modules process information in their compartments. Compartments communicate with other compartments in the same module, and with compartments in other modules.

The central module

A module, which will be called here the central module, integrates information from all the other modules. As a result, information structures that span across modules are formed. For example, each of the cars that head into each other in the example mentioned earlier is represented by a node in the central module. All the properties of each of the cars, as represented by nodes in peripheral modules, are parts of the corresponding node in the central module. Information about the motion of the cars may reach the feeling module, and evoke feelings about the simulated event. The feelings and the peripheral stimuli, as well as other associated events can be accessed and manipulated by the central module.

The central module contains also nodes that fire on their own. These nodes represent the activities that start from within the system, such as those of the autonomic nervous system, and the innate drives. The latter are of special interest here, and will be discussed in a later chapter. These nodes may be affected by inputs from other nodes, including peripheral stimuli, but they maintain a core of independence in their operation.

A CPU can handle interrupts. After receiving an interrupt, a CPU will divert its activities and execute another program, as indicated by the interrupt. After completing that program, the CPU may resume its old routine, or do something else. The CPU scans interrupt ports regularly, and when a flag indicates that an interrupt request has arrived, the CPU responds appropriately. The brain also recognizes interrupts, and the model can handle them. In the model, interrupts reach the central module, where they are evaluated. The identification of an activation-pattern as a warranted interrupt is done in the appropriate module, which then sends an interrupt signal to the central module. Based on the status of the entire system, as represented in the central module, a response is chosen. For example, a ring of a doorbell or of a telephone are processed and recognized as justified interrupts by the auditory module, which forwards an interrupt instruction to the central module. The central module may then evaluate the state of the entire system and may instruct appropriate modules to stop their ongoing activity and start a different one.

In general, all the modules process information concurrently, within their perimeter. When the processed information involves a number of modules, the information converges to the central unit, where it is processed, and from where it is relayed to other modules.

3. MODULES IN THE BRAIN AND IN THE MODEL

The various modules share common operation and design principles, and at the same time, they maintain some module-specific characteristics. In the following, the visual module will serve as the prototype for describing the structural elements and the main operation principles of peripheral modules. The general characteristics of some inner modules will then be outlined. More details about information handling by the modules are given in subsequent chapters.

Representing classes and items

The lens of the eye projects an image of the three-dimensional outside world onto the two-dimensional retina, at the back of the eye. The retina can be divided into imaginary small pixels, which, from a practical point of view, are the smallest elements that make up the entire picture. In the pixels of the retina, light sensing neurons–the rods and the cones–convert incoming light stimuli into electrical pulses. Processing of these signals starts at the retina itself. From there, signals are forwarded directly and indirectly to other parts of the brain, including the primary visual cortex, where neurons are organized in columns. These columns receive pulses that are associated with the same pixel of the retina. Thus, the pixel can serve as the labeling address of the column. Different neurons at the same cortical column are fired by different feature combinations that involve their labeling pixel. Hence, these neurons represent different feature combinations that are associated with their pixel. The outside world is mapped onto the retina, and this topographic representation is preserved to certain extent in the arrangement of the directly affected cortical columns. Neighboring elements of an observed object activate neighboring retinal pixels, which activate neurons in neighboring columns. The cortical columns can also receive stimuli from other parts of the brain, including from other visual cortex areas.

Then, neurons in different columns, each of which can be labeled by its own retinal pixel, send their outputs to neurons in other columns, further away in the cortex. Neurons in the latter columns receive stimuli that have originated at different retinal pixels. Thus, they represent feature combinations of several pixels. The complexity of these feature combinations increases as we move further into the cortex. The simplest feature combinations contain information about the pixel itself, such as the intensity and color of its illumination. Then come combinations that involve the pixel and its adjacent surroundings, such as bright center with dark surrounding, or the opposite. Next in complexity are combinations of illuminated lines that contain the pixel. These lines can be of different lengths and widths, and they can be stationary or in motion. A neuron that fires when a certain bar of light illuminates a specific group of retinal pixel plays the role of an item-node. It represents the specific bar as a whole, and the illuminated pixels are represented by its part-nodes.

In addition to neurons that play the role of item-nodes, there are neurons that represent events that are not associated with any specific pixel. For example, some neurons fire when a certain bar of light illuminates any part of the retina. Such neurons play the role of class-nodes. Their exemplars are all those nodes that represent that bar of light at a specific location in the retina. As the bar of light moves across the field of view, it activates those exemplar-nodes one at a time. Each of these exemplar-nodes, in turn, activates their common class-node.

As the signals continue to propagate to other cortical regions, neurons there integrate the activities from many columns or, equivalently, from larger fields of view of the outside world, and express them as related items, parts, exemplars, and classes.

This general architecture, which repeats itself in brain areas of other senses, is the motivation to the various modules presented here, and their interacting compartments. The neurons of the input pixel and of the cortical columns are represented in the model by the pixel's-clusters of the arena. They represent the basic features of the module that the model can handle.

Detectors and projectors

Detectors of an arena, such as line detectors, are those nodes that are activated by specific combinations of features that appear in the pixel's-clusters. An arena has many detectors, and they can process information simultaneously. Some detectors observe the sensors directly, while some get their inputs from other detectors.

The projectors of a module are neurons that send signals in the reverse direction, and activate detector neurons or neurons in pixel's-clusters. By so doing, they simulate events in the arena. Projectors may be initiated by neurons in the same module or by neurons from other modules. Neurons in the speech and hearing modules are important initiators of projectors in other modules. It is plausible to assume that when we hear the word 'cat', neurons in the speech and hearing modules cause the activation of neurons in the visual arena, which represent visual clues of a specific cat or of cats in general.

The various detectors and projectors constitute the basic building blocks for the concepts that the system employs. The detectors determine which feature combinations in the peripheral stimuli will be looked for, and, when found, will be used to describe and to relate to the environment. Similarly, the projectors determine which feature combinations will be used in the simulation of the environment at the arena, so that the system will be able to evaluate its responses to external situations without actually executing them.

The circuitry of some detectors and the projectors is innate, while others acquire it through experience. Both kinds participate in processing the data in the module.

Common operations in modules

Parsing and clustering, sameness

A large number of retinal pixels are stimulated concurrently, as they represent the outside world. This group of firing neurons is parsed by the detectors of the module. Edge detectors provide means for dividing a big scene into sub-scenes. Abrupt changes in any feature represented by neurons in the pixel's-cluster may indicate where the large scene should be divided into sub-scenes. Such sub-scenes, in turn, are clustered into hierarchies of items and their parts. For example, after a given scene that contains a house is parsed into areas of similar characteristics, those areas are clustered into a hierarchy of items and parts such as the whole house, its windows, its walls and their bricks, its door and its doorknob etc.

A scene may be parsed by mechanisms other than edge detection. For example, firing neurons that represent the same feature in neighboring pixels may recruit another neuron to represent them as its parts, thus defining an item. This may explain how a line of any shape, drawn on a piece of paper, is perceived as one object. First, the points of that line stimulate the same-feature detector in neighboring pixel's-columns. Then, all these stimulated neurons recruit another neuron to represent them as one item.

From an operational point of view, the process of parsing and clustering is based on two sub-processes: detecting relevant criteria and actually using them in the clustering. A firing neuron indicates the presence of a feature that may serve as a clustering criterion. The notion that different firing neurons, which belong to different pixels, can represent the **same** feature is crucial to the clustering process. This **sameness** of features has to be embedded in the network. In this model, the class-exemplar relationship is used to represent sameness of features. All the nodes that represent the same feature are exemplars of the same class, which is represented by its own node. For example, nodes that represent the green color of their corresponding pixels are exemplars of the class 'green'. This class is represented by its own node, which relates to all the 'green' nodes as its exemplars. A pattern of firing pixels that possess the same feature could be represented by the part-item relationship. Those pixels would recruit a node to represent them. This node would be the item-node, and the feature nodes would be its parts. For example, when a group of retinal pixels is stimulated by green light (such as a patch of green grass in a scene) all the firing green nodes in the pixel's-clusters can recruit a node to represent them. They would be the parts, and the recruited node would be the item, which is the green patch in the scene.

Each pixel's-cluster has one node, which represents the pixel itself, and a number of nodes that represent various properties of that pixel-node. The connections between those nodes would vary from module to module, and even within the same module. Figure 3.1 shows three hypothetical pixels and their features, arranged in pixel's-clusters. One of the features possessed by every pixel's-cluster is 'green'. To encode the sameness of that feature, these feature-nodes are made to be exemplars of the class node 'green'. When the color of a retinal pixel is green, its corresponding 'green' node in the pixel's-cluster fires. Assume now that in a given scene the two leftmost pixels are green. They will be represented by the firing green nodes in the two leftmost pixel's-clusters. These firing nodes may recruit a node to represent them as a green item in the field of view.

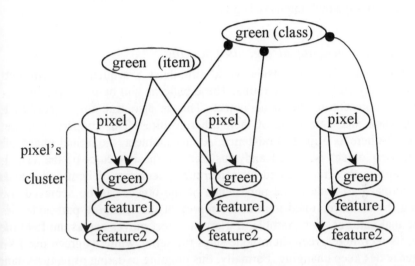

Figure 3.1: Three pixels and their pixel's-clusters. The sameness of the feature green is represented by all the green nodes in the clusters being exemplars of one class node–green. If in a certain event, the two leftmost pixels are green, their firing green features may become parts of a recruited green item.

While the sameness of some features is innately embedded in the network, the system is capable of determining whether two new items are the same, meaning **identical** to each other, or not. Sameness detectors can determine if two items that appear at the same time in different parts of the arena are the same. In addition, detectors can also determine if a real item and a memory item are the same. If a real item that is active due to external stimulation does not have a corresponding same memory item, the real item is **new**.

Comparing features

The most fundamental group of detectors in the visual module are those that detect the color and the brightness of a single retinal pixel. They can also detect time variations of these features. Next, come detectors that compare properties of two retinal pixels. They detect if the pixels have the same color or not. They can also detect if there are intensity differences between the two pixels, and if so, which intensity is greater.

Object-persistence, appearing, disappearing

A moving object in the outside world stimulates a sequence of different neural activity patterns in the retina. These patterns will be perceived by the brain as representing the same object. This is also true for objects that change their shape or some of their other features. This property will be referred to here as **object-persistence**. At any moment, the retinal image of the moving object is parsed and clustered by the detectors of the visual arena, and is thus represented by a recruited hierarchy of item-nodes and their retinal part-nodes. The persistence of the object can be achieved by having the same recruited item-nodes represent the changing part-nodes in the retinal patterns. For example, if a green object moves across the field of view, its recruited 'green' item-node stays the same, while its green pixel's-cluster nodes keep changing. Formally, this ongoing updating of features can be accomplished by the use of the basic dissociation and association operations. Old green pixels are dissociated from the item-node, while new ones become associated to it. According to this view, any firing node in a pixel's-cluster indicates the presence of its feature as a part of the item. It also represents the location, or **coordinate**, of that feature in a retinal coordinate system. The coordinates of all these pixels constitute the coordinates of the item. Coordinates of an item are its parts. These coordinates may change with time without the item losing its identity.

The module has also detectors that detect the **appearance** of new objects and the disappeance of old ones in the arena. What is perceived as one moving object, as opposed to one object that disappears at one point and another similar object that appears at a nearby point, depends on the intrinsic properties of those detectors. If the second object appears before the first has completely faded out, the two objects may be perceived as one moving object.

Detecting the common

Common detectors identify groups of nodes that belong to two or more items. Since only contiguous parts of an item are automatically activated when the item-node is activated, common detectors have mechanisms to compare the explicated parts of the involved items.

Operating in parallel

Many detectors operate simultaneously in the arena, and they can analyze different items. To be useful, detected properties have to be associated with the appropriate items and the appropriate procedure. For example, if car A is moving to the right and car B is moving to the left, the detected properties 'moving to the right' and 'moving to the left' have to be associated with the appropriate cars. Such associations are carried out by forming connections between corresponding nodes. The system has means to mark activated nodes according to the procedure in which they participate. That marking enables the system to process information in parallel.

Projecting mental pictures

Fundamental properties, which are detectable by the detectors, can also be projected onto the arena by the projectors. Very often, in order to solve a problem, the projectors generate its mental picture in the arena. This mental picture is then analyzed by the detectors. For example, to answer the question 'how many intersections (common points) can two straight lines have?' various straight-line configurations are first projected onto the visual arena. These projections are then analyzed by the detectors of the arena. The outcome of this analysis provides the grounds for our answer.

Projectors activate nodes in the arena so that they simulate elements of real world situations. The projectors establish links, which connect the activated nodes of the arena with item-nodes that are the subject of the simulation. For example, to create a mental picture of 'a red car moves to the right', a pattern of pixel's-clusters nodes that represent 'red car' are selected and activated. These nodes are connected as parts to an item-node that represents the 'red car'. This item-node is also an exemplar of the class 'red car'. As such, it inherits properties that are common to all the red cars. The projector then 'moves' to the right of the arena the part-nodes that represent 'red car', in a way that preserve the object-persistence of the item-node 'red car', as explained earlier. All these activated nodes form a mental picture of a red car moving to the right. The images can be analyzed by the detectors, and provide various consequences of the mental event. Like detectors, projectors operate in parallel, and can establish connections between the appropriate nodes.

Other peripheral modules

The auditory, somatosensory, vestibular, olfactory, and taste modules have some structure and operation principles similar to those of the visual module, although the information that they encode and process has different meanings. Except for the olfactory module, the spatial distributions of the physical peripheral sensors are mapped onto parts of the cortex. There, columns of neurons represent different properties of pixels in the sensory areas. These pixels can serve as labels of the neural columns. Neighboring columns usually represent events that occur in neighboring pixels, with a certain amount of overlapping. This arrangement is represented in the module by the arenas and their pixel's-clusters. The nodes in the pixel's-clusters represent the most fundamental concepts of their module. Processing of the data is carried out by detectors, which extract specific feature combinations that are present in the input patterns, and assemble them into the more complex concepts of the module. These assembled concepts are represented by nodes further up in the module. Projectors can project events onto the arenas and simulate real events.

The entire surface of the body is mapped onto the somatosensory cortex. Body regions, such as fingers, which require higher resolution in sensing their inputs, are represented by larger numbers of neurons in the somatosensory cortex, while body regions that require less resolution, like the back, are represented by relatively less neurons. Each cortical column contains neurons that are connected to different sensors such as pressure, pain, heat, cold, and some chemical sensors. The firing of these neurons indicate the presence of these features at their pixels.

Sounds that enter the ear cause patterns of mechanical vibrations of the basilar membrane in the cochlea. These vibrations are picked up by hair-cell sensors, whose locations label the frequencies, and whose electric output encode the intensities of their particular basilar pixel. Like the rods and the cones of the eye, each hair-cell in the cochlea is most sensitive to a certain frequency, but it responds also to other frequencies. The electric signals propagate from the hair-cells directly and indirectly to other parts of the brain, including the auditory cortex. Columns of neurons represent feature combinations of sound that involve the same pixel of the basilar membrane. All these principles are modeled by the sound module. Pixel's-cluster nodes represent feature combinations that involve their pixel. Detectors of the arena detect various properties and spatial and temporal correlations of activated pixels. These detected features are assembled into hierarchies of items and parts, which are the concepts of the auditory module.

Details of the topographic distribution of the chemical senses and the encoding systems that they utilize are less known than those of the other modules. It is plausible to assume that here too, complex concepts are formed from basic ones. They are represented and can be projected in the module like the concepts in the other modules.

The motor module is one of the peripheral modules. Unlike the sensory modules just mentioned, the arena of the motor module contains also output elements. These neurons initiate activities in the muscles and glands. The detailed mechanisms by which the brain controls and coordinates the activities of the muscles are complex and are still under investigation. Columns of neurons in the motor cortex map the various body parts, similarly to the neurons of the somatosensory cortex. Stimulation of neurons in the motor cortex results in the activation of their corresponding muscles. However, many other parts of the brain are involved in controlling muscle activities. For the sake of simplicity, this model will assume that the arena of the motor module contains activation pixels, which activate individual muscles. Each pixel has its own pixel's-cluster, which represents various activation modes of that individual muscle. In addition, each pixel's-cluster has sensory neurons, which monitor the actual state of the muscle and represent them. The motor module has detectors that characterize spatio-temporal activation and status patterns of individual muscles. The motor module has projectors that can simulate such patterns in the motor arena.

Inner modules

Inner modules receive their input from other modules and process it. They have arenas, detectors, and projectors like the peripheral modules. Their detectors identify and represent specific feature combinations as whole-parts and exemplar-classes hierarchies. Thus, they form additional concepts, according to which the system represents and analyzes the self and the environment. Following is a general description of some inner modules.

Inter-sensory association modules

Association areas in the brain include intra-modality and inter-modality areas such as visual-auditory, visual-motor, and auditory-motor association areas. Like association areas within a module, association modules integrate information from different modules. They manipulate representations of non-fundamental concepts that have been formed in other modules. Therefore, the meanings of their own input-pixels are not innate. Input nodes in these arenas are recruited to represent concept of other modules. Integrated concepts from different modules are then represented in the association module as item-part and class-exemplar hierarchies. Projectors of the module can activate these integrated concepts in the association module as well as their sources in the other modules.

The feeling module

As sensory neurons provide information about external physical conditions, the brain needs to evaluate what is good and what is bad for the body. This is done at the feeling module. Input from peripheral modules reaches the feeling module, and activates innate detectors that detect and expresses various desirable, benign, and noxious situations. These detectors are innate to the system. Some of them have innate connections that lead all the way to pixels of peripheral arenas. For example, the noxious feeling that 'the finger is squeezed' is initiated by the activation of innately-connected peripheral pressure sensors of the finger, which are found in the somatosensory arena. Signals from the squeezed finger reach the feeling module and activate a noxious-detector, which creates the perception that the squeezed finger is a noxious situation.

In addition to being innately defined and wired, nodes of the feeling module can develop new ties and represent and record learned episodes that the system has experienced. Like other modules, the feeling module has detectors that detect and represent temporal characteristics of the fundamental concepts. These include certain qualifiers of feelings such as: has just started, is ongoing, is increasing or decreasing in magnitude, or has ended.

All the desirable feelings are exemplars of a node that represents the concept 'desirable'. Similarly, there is a node that represents the class 'noxious', whose exemplars are the various noxious feelings. Another class node represents the class 'benign', whose exemplar nodes represent specific benign feelings. Many of the sensations that cause the various feelings are initiated by well-identified sensors at the somatosensory module. However, there are feelings whose neural initiators are difficult to pinpoint, e.g. being in love (no, it does not start at the heart...). Initiators of such feelings are spread over the entire system. For the sake of convenience, the model will represent them by virtual nodes at the feeling module. These nodes will be activated by nodes at other modules. As more becomes known about those activating nodes, the information could be incorporated into the model in the form of standard connections between the initiator nodes and the feeling node. The sensations of love, hate, anger, hunger, thirst, fatigue, freshness, joy, sadness, fear, safety, anticipation, and the likes could be treated as fundamental feeling concepts, until more is known about their neural circuitries.

The output of the feeling module characterizes the feeling that its input has caused. This output may serve as input to other modules, which have to decide on a response, or on recording in memory the novel experience and its consequences.

The communication module

Language is one of the means that humans use to communicate with each other. Animals, too, use sound, body language, and other means to exchange information. In communication, the original message, which is represented by a pattern of firing neurons, invokes an associated neural representation of a sound, a posture, or something of similar nature. The latter activate corresponding motor units that broadcast the coded message. On the other end, in the receiver's system, sensory modules detect and analyze the communicated code. They then activate an associated pattern of neurons, which are the representation of the original message in the receiver's system. The receiver's system can then analyze that pattern, and act upon it.

When sending a message out, the responsibility of a human communication module is to encode the original message in a lingual format, and then to activate the appropriate motor units that transmit it. When receiving a message, the communication module is responsible to capture the lingual code and to translate it into its original format, so that it could be used by the system.

Some communication processes are innate and some are learned. For example, screaming as a result of a sudden scare seems to be executed by innate circuitry. Courtship displays in some bird species may also be driven by innate circuitry. However, most of the messages communicated by humans are not innate.

Humans have a very elaborate and flexible communication system that can encode neural activation patterns into lingual expressions. The lingual expressions can be in auditory (spoken) or visual (written) formats. Animals are apparently using simpler, less flexible, and more direct encoding systems.

In the model, the communication module will have to rely on a variety of operation units, because many details of its operations are not known yet. However, the module would have nodes that represent concepts in their lingual form. Those nodes would be connected to each other by the standard connections of the model, which represent exemplar-class and item-part relationships. These relationships may duplicate the relationships of their original concepts. For example, 'dog' is an exemplar of the class 'animal'. This class-exemplar relationship may be realized by nodes in the communication module and by nodes in peripheral modules that represent past experiences.

The central module

The central module is an association module that can associate information from all other modules. Its item nodes may have parts that are directly connected with nodes in other modules. They can also be exemplars of classes in other modules. This makes it possible for nodes at certain modules to inherit properties from nodes at other modules. The nodes of the central module are often recruited for limited tasks, and when the task is over, they are de-commissioned. Thinking operations that depend on information from many modules are coordinated by the central module, which can also record events that involve other modules. Awareness also takes place in the central module. Being aware of states and processes that occur in other modules is represented by awareness nodes, which reside in the central module.

4. THE BASIC CONCEPTS

Types of concepts and their representations

Words encapsulate concepts that we use to parse and describe situations in our world. Language, by combining words, relies on simple concepts to describe a variety of complex situations. The same situations that are described by the language are also represented by patterns of firing neurons in the brain. It may be said that in addition to describing the world, language describes patterns of activated neurons in our brain. These patterns may be regarded as an "internal language", used by the brain to describe the world. Certain patterns of activated neurons play the role of "words" in this "internal language" of the brain.

Patterns of activated neurons are not mapped one-to-one into words. Many activated patterns are not represented by words, and very often, a word would represent various patterns, depending on its context in the sentence. However, it seems that many words have corresponding patterns of activated neurons, which are the elements of the brain's "internal language".

In the model presented here, a node represents a neuron or a group of neurons. So, the "internal language" of the brain can be expressed by patterns of activated nodes. In some cases, individual nodes represent situations that can be expressed lingually. In other cases, the whole pattern of nodes may have lingual correlates, while its individual nodes have no such correlate.

In the model, a concept that is represented by an entire pattern will also be represented by one equivalent concept-node. When that pattern is present, the concept-node will fire, and vice versa. When a pattern activates its concept-node, the latter acts as a detector. In a projection operation, the concept-node is activated first and its firing causes the activation of the pattern that it represents. This is a simulation of a real event, and it is used in thinking processes. In retrieval, the concept-node is activated according to a

51

cue, which is a pattern of active nodes that are associated with the retrieved node.

The model assumes that there is a small group of **innate concepts** from which all the other **acquired concepts** are composed. An acquired concept can be decomposed to an equivalent network of innate concepts that are interconnected by the standard connections.

There are two kinds of innate concepts: **innate atomic concepts** and **innate relational concepts**. Atomic concepts do not have parts that are concepts in the system. They are represented by nodes that are directly activated by factors from outside of the system. For example, an illuminated point in the field of view is considered an innate atomic concept. It is stimulated by external light sources. The sensation of hunger is another example of an innate atomic concept. It is caused by certain chemicals or by the lack thereof in the body.

Some innate concepts are represented by two **coupled nodes**—a sensor node and its internal representation node. The purpose of this arrangement is to be able to distinguish between a physical sensation and the thought about it. When the sensor node is stimulated by an external factor, it automatically activates its coupled internal node. The sensor node cannot be activated by internal factors. On the other hand, the internal node can be activated by internal factors and by the sensor node, but it cannot activate the sensor node. When we feel hunger, the sensor-node is activated and activates its coupled internal node. When we think about hunger, the coupled internal node is activated, but it does not activate the sensor node. Sensor nodes are activated only in detection operation, while their coupled nodes are activated in detection, projection, and retrieval operations.

Relational concepts can be innate or acquired. A relational concept is represented by a node that fires when certain relationships exist between other firing nodes. In addition to the representing node, a relational concept has two main parts: variable nodes that activate its representing node, and an inner circuitry that connects the variable nodes to the representing node. For example, the concept of a moving point of light is an innate relational concept. A neuron that fires when a point of light moves across the retina represents the relational concept 'a moving point of light'. Its variable nodes are the firing neurons of the retina that detect the presence of that light at different locations at different times. The inner circuitry makes the representing neuron fire as the point of light is moving across the retina.

A concept may be binary or multi-valued. An active node that represents a binary concept indicates its presence in the scene. When the binary node is quiet, the concept is absent from the scene. Multi-valued concepts are represented in biological networks by neurons that may have a variety of temporal firing patterns. For example, the rate of firing of a pressure sensor increases with the applied pressure. In the model, a multi-valued concept is represented by a group of mutually exclusive binary nodes, each of which representing a range of values. When all these nodes are quiet, the concept is absent from the current scene. Otherwise, only one of the binary nodes can be active at any given time, indicating the value of the concept. All these binary nodes are exemplars of a class node, whose firing represents the presence of the concept, without specifying its value.

Some concepts are very prevalent in the environment, while others are quite rare. A set of concepts that can be used to express all other concepts will be referred to as a set of **basic concepts**. The set of basic concepts consists of innate and acquired concepts that may be prevalent or rare. It may be possible to express some of the basic concepts by others. The benefit of such a redundancy is efficiency in the representation. If a complex basic concept contains a combination of many simpler ones, when using the complex concept to represent another concept there is no need to spell out all those simpler concepts that it contains.

The model's initial concepts

The brain has a set of innate concepts with which it starts to operate. It uses them to process its experiences, and consequently it acquires new concepts. It keeps processing new experiences based on the accumulated concepts, while adding newly developed concepts to its repertoire. Like the brain, the model starts with an initial set of given concepts. It keeps expanding and using its concepts according to its operation rules and its experiences. The initial concepts determine how new experiences are decomposed and perceived by the model. They also determine the limitations of the model–which details of events could never be grasped by the model.

Some of the brain's innate concepts and many of its acquired ones are well known, but it is still debatable whether certain concepts are innate or acquired. Because of that and because of other practical reasons, the initial concepts that the model relies upon would not necessarily be the innate concepts of the brain. Rather, those concepts would be determined by the intended scope of the model. The basic concepts include some obvious innate brain concepts such as various fundamental sensory stimuli. Other basic concepts are common elementary concepts, whose nature can be inferred by observing the behavior of the entire system. The purpose of the model is to demonstrate how all the concepts function as an ensemble, even if the biological mechanisms of some individual concepts are not known. By so doing, the model parses the domain of unknown brain-mechanisms into sub-domains, which might be easier to tackle experimentally.

A chosen set of basic concepts can always be expanded by adding new concepts. It is also possible to replace a basic concept by a structure of concepts, especially when it becomes clear how to represent an acquired concept by innate ones. The rest of this chapter describes a set of basic concepts, and illustrates some of the derived concepts that can be constructed from them. Many brain activities can be expressed by these concepts, but in order to represent all possible activities of the brain, additional basic and derived concepts would have to be added.

A model that could describe all the activities of the brain should have all the basic concepts that the brain may use. Compiling such a list and proving its completeness is a daunting task that still has to be done. The rest of the chapter introduces a partial list of various kinds of basic concepts, showing how they can be incorporated into the model.

The basic atomic concepts

The basic atomic nodes that the model uses do not always correspond to receptor-cells in biological systems. For example, the sensation of the color of a retinal pixel is determined by three different kinds of light receptors, which are found in that pixel. The illumination at neighboring pixels may also contribute to that sensation. The model represents the color of a pixel by a single multi-valued node. Each value corresponds to one of the thousands of colors that we can perceive. The details of the biological mechanisms of color perception at the receptor level are beyond the scope of the model. Another example is the sensation of taste. The four major taste sensations of salty, sour, bitter, and sweet have identifiable taste-bud receptors. However, a taste receptor would usually respond to more than one of these tastes, and the many flavors that we can recognize are determined by the simultaneous activities of different taste and smell receptors. Thus, if the model employs a dedicated node to represent 'vanilla' as a basic taste sensation, it does not intend to imply that there is a specialized receptor neuron for the vanilla flavor.

When constructing a brain model, it is possible to choose its basic concepts in many different ways, because the basic concepts do not necessarily correspond one-to-one with individual neurons. In the following, sets of basic concepts for various modules are suggested. These sets have been assembled so that a large number of concepts could be constructed from them. Other sets of basic concepts could probably achieve that same goal. In general, the basic concepts of a model have to be chosen so that it would be possible to express with them all the concepts that the model has to handle.

Visual module

The main atomic concepts of the visual arena are organized in pixel's-clusters. The 'point' node (figure 4.1) represents the corresponding pixel, or

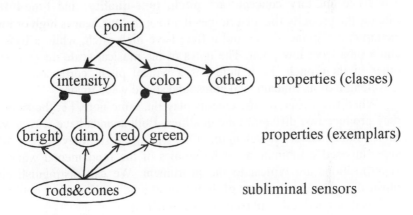

Figure 4.1: Possible organization of a visual pixel's-cluster.

point, in the retina. 'Point' is a basic concept. It has part-nodes, which represent its properties. The synaptic weights between the 'intensity' and 'color' nodes and the 'point' node are such that only when those two part nodes are present together, the item node 'point' fires. The two part nodes–

'color' and 'color intensity'–are also basic concepts. They have their own exemplars, representing various colors and various illumination intensities at the point. All these nodes have connections with other nodes in the system. Through these connections, they can participate in various system activities. On the other hand, nodes that represent the rods and cones of the biological retina are 'subliminal'. They affect the pixel's-cluster nodes that represent the actual color and color-intensity of the pixel, but they themselves cannot be accessed by the rest of the system. The are represented in the model by computation units.

All the input pixels of the visual arena have this same structure. The sameness property of corresponding elements of different pixels is expressed in the model by the class-exemplar relationship. As discussed above, all the nodes that represent the 'same' properties at different pixels, (e.g. 'green' as in figure 3.1), are exemplar of the same class node. They can be accessed by other nodes of the system.

Auditory module

The basic auditory concepts are **pitch, tone-quality**, and **tone-intensity**. Pitch is the property that determines if a tone that we hear is high or low. For example, a soprano singer and a flute have high pitch, while a bass singer and a tuba have low pitch. The notes of the musical scale differ from each other in their pitch. Each note has a typical pitch, corresponding to the wavelength of its fundamental sinusoidal sound wave in air.

When two different instruments play the same note, i.e. the same pitch, they produce two different tone qualities. Both sounds have waves with the same fundamental wavelength. On top of that, they have different superimposed combinations of harmonics of the fundamental wave. Those superpositions are typical to the instrument. We can distinguish between musical instruments because of their typical tone-qualities (has nothing to do with bad or good tones, players, or instruments).

Tone intensity is how strong or weak a sound is. It depends on the amplitude of the sound waves.

The different pitches are the pixel nodes of the auditory module. Each pixel has its own pixel's-cluster, with many nodes. Every node in the pixel's-cluster is multi-valued, and it represents one tone-quality. The different intensities of any tone-quality are represented by its tone-intensity node. One of the nodes in the pixel's-cluster represents the total intensity of its pitch, regardless of which tone-qualities are present. Figure 4.2 illustrates a typical auditory pixel's-cluster. It shows only the nodes that are handled by the model. It does not show nodes that represent actual auditory sensors. These are subliminal to the model, and they activate all the appropriate nodes of the pixel's-cluster as needed. They can be represented by computation units.

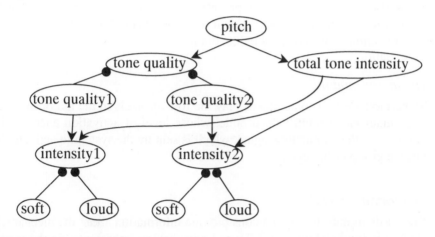

Figure 4.2: Some nodes of auditory pixel's-cluster. Subliminal nodes are not shown.

While pitch is usually used to label sounds that consist of one fundamental wavelength, its use can be extended in the model to describe other sounds. Any sound, such as the sound of a spoken word, is a superposition of sound waves of different wavelengths. The model can consider each spoken word or each phoneme as an extended pitch, which has its own node. Similar to musical instrument, the voice of any speaking individual can be characterized by its tone quality and intensity. These, too, will have their own nodes. Thus, the selection of the set of fundamental 'pitches', 'tone-qualities', and 'intensities' can be determined by the situations that have to be handled by the auditory module in the model.

Somatic (bodily) module

The surface of the body is divided into pixels of sensory spots. Each spot has a pixel's-cluster of nodes, which describe various types of basic sensations that can be felt at the pixel. These include **touch, warmth, cold,** and **pain.**

Each of these sensations is a multi-valued concept, which is represented by a node in the pixel's-cluster. Nodes of the same sensation (e.g. touch) that belong to different pixels are exemplars of a class-node that represents that sensation. There is not a one-to-one correspondence between these basic sensations and biological receptors. Neurons along various pathways from the skin all the way to the brain process somatosensory information. Signals from these neurons and from the skin receptors themselves determine how a somatic stimulus is perceived by the brain.

The motor module

Muscle groups and some glands play the role of pixels in the motor module. Each pixel has a multi-valued node, whose level of activation encodes the intensity of the stimulating signal, which is sent by the system to activate the muscle group or the gland.

The posture module

Receptors in muscles and tendons provide information about the mechanical state of individual body parts. These body parts are represented in the model as basic pixel nodes, whose pixel's-clusters represent the sensations felt in them. These include the activity states of **relax, stretch, contract,** and **muscle pain** for skeletal muscles, and **strain** and **internal pain** sensations for other internal organs. Vestibular receptors sense the **orientation** of the head with respect to the Earth. They also sense when the head is **accelerated, decelerated,** or **rotated**. These vestibular sensations, which are basic concepts, are multi-valued in their intensities and cover all the range of possible orientations of the head in space.

The taste and smell module

The basic concepts of this module are all the different stimuli that we can recognize as individual tastes and odors. Some of these entities are related to others through the class-exemplar relationship. For example, the model considers sweet to be a basic taste concept. The tastes of honey and sugar are two basic taste concepts, which are exemplars of the class sweet. Some familiar taste concepts can be defined as combinations of basic concepts e.g. 'sweet and sour'.

The feeling module

Innate feelings about the state of the body are the basic concepts of the feeling module. These feelings are divided into three major classes: **pleasant, benign**, and **unpleasant**. Each of the feeling nodes is an exemplar of one of those classes. These exemplars may reside in the feeling module, or they may be real or virtual nodes in other modules. They become activated by patterns of firing neurons that represent states of the system that cause the corresponding feeling. The details of these activator patterns could be implemented in the model by the standard connections of the model, once they are explored in biological systems. Here is a partial list of these feelings, each represented by its own node: **comfort, discomfort, happy, joy, sad, safe, fear, hunger, thirst, sate, fresh, tired, awake, sleepy, alert, numb, excited, calm, sober, intoxicated, interested, bored, curious, familiar, novel, apathetic,** various **sexual drives and sexual sensations, sensations of the digestive** and **the cardiovascular** systems, **love, hate, anger.**

The central module

An important group of basic concepts of the central module are those that represent mental and awareness processes and states. They include various thinking processes and their sub-processes such as **searching for a solution, having a potential solution, evaluating a potential solution, approval of a solution, having found a partial solution, and recording data.** Concepts that deal with state of mind and awareness such as **imagining, day dreaming, dreaming, wanting, anticipating,** being **aware of**, and being in **control of** these and all other nodal activities are also concepts represented at the central module.

Basic relational concepts and constructors

The basic relational concepts enable the system to combine simpler concepts into more complex ones, and to decompose complex concepts into their more fundamental elements. As concepts, relational concepts can appear as detectors and as projectors. In the brain, their activities may be carried out by entire circuitries, but in the model, many of them are represented by single nodes or by operation units. The reason is that we do not know all the details of the biological structure and the mechanisms that are employed by the brain. The only thing that we do know is that the brain uses them. It is left to the simulation program to replicate the effects of the inputs of relational concepts on the representing nodes, which represent the relational concepts to the rest of the system.

Definitions and notations

Relational concepts encode specific relationships that exist between other concepts. Some relational concepts represent the same type of relationship in different modules, while others are module specific. In general, a relational concept can be expressed as a triad of the form (A, relation, B), where concepts 'A' and 'B' may be variables, and 'relation' is the particular relational concept. A relational concept can be multi-valued when any of its variables is multi-valued.

In a **symmetric** relational concept, the concept (A, relation, B) is the same as (B, relation, A) for any two concepts 'A' and 'B', e.g. (A,is-identical-to,B). In an **asymmetric** relational concept, (A, relation, B) is different from (B, relation, A), e.g. (A, is-brighter-than,B).

In a **transitive** relational concept, the situations (A,transitive-relation,B) and (B,transitive-relation,C) implies the situation (A,transitive-relation,C). This property of transitive relations is embedded in the system. For example, (A,greater,B) and (B,greater,C) guarantees that (A,greater,C) holds too in the system.

When the concept operates as a projector, its firing representing node activates its variable nodes. Those activated nodes can be detected by the detectors of the system. For example, if 'A', 'B', and 'C' are projected such that 'A' is greater than 'B' and 'B' is greater than 'C', the detectors will detect that 'A' is greater than 'C' even though this relationship was not projected explicitly.

A boldface variable, such as '**A**', indicates a group of nodes. The notation (**A**,relation,B) indicates that each member of the group '**A**' is related to 'B' through 'relation'. The notation (**A**,relation,**B**) indicates that there is a one-to-one mapping between groups '**A**' and '**B**', and that mapped pairs are related through 'relation'.

The following notations will be used in order to distinguish between the various modes in which relational concepts operate in the system:

- The notation (A, relation, B) indicates that a structure that represents 'A', 'B' and the fact that they satisfy 'relation' is projected in the appropriate module.

A question mark attached to the expression indicates that the concept acts as a detector or as a cue.

- The notation (A, relation, B)? indicates that 'relation' acts as a detector–when events 'A' and 'B' that possess the particular relationship are present, the node that represents that relationship fires.
- The expression (?,relation,B) indicates that 'A' has to be retrieved when 'relation' and 'B' are specified. Similarly, the following are other possible cues: (A,relation,?), (A,?,B), (?,relation,?).
- The notation (?A,relation,B?) indicates a query that checks if (A, relation, B) is true or false. 'A' and 'B' are provided as variables to 'relation', and if 'relation' fires, the answer to the query is yes. Otherwise, the answer is no.
- A missing parameter, such as (,relation,B), indicates that the relation does not depend on that parameter.

In addition to detecting and projecting relational concepts in their arenas, events that contain relational concepts have to be recorded in the memory. When a relational concept operates as a detector, it analyzes properties of the participating concepts, and determines if the particular relationship exists between them. It may be advantageous for the system to record the outcome of such an analysis, so that in the future it won't be necessary to repeat it. Whenever those concepts recur, the system could use the recorded information to indicate that they satisfy the particular relationship, without going again through the analysis. One possible mechanism of recording relational concepts is the following (illustrated in figure 4.3): Assume that concepts 'A' and 'B' satisfy relationship 'relation1', and they have just activated the detector (A,relation1,B)?. This prompts the recording process. First, 'A' and 'B' recruit an item node to represent them as its parts. Then, this item node becomes an exemplar of the class node 'records of relation1', whose exemplars are combinations, like 'A and B', that have activated 'relation1'. The class-node 'records of relation1' has its own parts, 'VAR1' and 'VAR2'. The node 'A' becomes an exemplar of 'VAR1', and node 'B' becomes an exemplar of 'VAR2'.

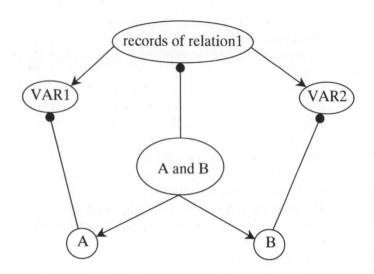

Figure 4.3: A memory record that stores the information that concepts 'A' and 'B' are related through the asymmetric relational concept 'relation1'. 'A' plays the role of the first variable of relation1, and 'B' plays the role of the second variable.

When 'A' and 'B' recur, the node 'records of relation1' fires, indicating that concepts 'A' and 'B' have been found in the past to satisfy the relational concept 'relation1'. This will not require to actually analyze the properties of 'A' and 'B'. The node 'records of relation1' acts as an **information detector**. It detects relationships between stored information entities, which are records of processed events. Question marks outside the parentheses of a concept indicate a query to the memory. For example, the notation ?(A,relation1,B)? is a query to an information detector. The detector will fire if there is a record in memory that concepts 'A' and 'B' possess relationship 'relation1'. If 'relation1' is an asymmetrical concept, the data structure of figure 4.3 makes it possible to identify the variables according to their roles in the relational concept. For example, if 'A is greater than B' is recorded, 'A' can be retrieved by the cue: an exemplar of 'VAR1' and a part of 'A and B'.

System-wide basic relational concepts

And/Or

The symmetric relational concept (A,and,B) expresses situations in which both concepts 'A' and 'B' are present. Let node 'C' represent the relational concept (A,and,B). The circuitry that connects these nodes is simple: Node 'C' is an item node, whose parts are nodes 'A' and 'B'. The item node 'C' inherits all the parts of its constituting concepts. As a detector, the concept-node 'A,and,B' fires when concepts 'A' and 'B' are present in the scene, or when the union of their parts is present. As a projector, it activates nodes 'A' and 'B'. To indicate that 'A' and 'B' form a new item, a node has to be recruited and 'A' and 'B' have to be connected to it as parts.

Similarly, the symmetric relational concept **or** pertains to situations where two or more concepts are exemplars of another real or virtual concept, which is their class node. As a detector, the concept-node 'A,or,B' fires when concept 'A' or concept 'B' are present in the scene. As a projector, it first projects concept 'A'. It then clears the scene and projects concept 'B'. For example, when we hear the forecast "It may rain or snow tomorrow", two scenes are projected in our mind one after the other: a scene of rain and a scene of snow.

Not

'Not' is a basic concept of set theory. Consider a set 'S' that one of its elements is 'A'. The statement 'not A' defines a subset of 'S', whose elements are all the elements of 'S' except the element 'A'. 'Not' is also a basic relational concept of the model. The node that represents the detector (,not,A)? fires when node 'A' is quiet and is quiet when node 'A' fires. This is in complete similarity to the conventions of set theory. However, from practical reasons, the projector (,not,A) does not activate all the nodes of the system except node 'A'. Instead, it inhibits node 'A' from firing. So, when (,not,A) is part of a projected scene, node 'A' will be quiet, while other nodes could be activated by other projectors. The absence of 'A' from the scene will be detected by a (,not,A) detector, which will fire as expected. In retrieving, the cue (,not,A) is an element of a wider retrieval request. It indicates that the concept 'A' cannot be a part the retrieved wider concept.

In human languages, the combination 'not A' is used quite often as a generic name for a concept that is the antonym of concept 'A'. The antonym may or may not have its own name. Consider the statement 'sticking out your tongue is not polite'. It indicates that the concept 'sticking out your tongue' is an exemplar of the class 'not polite', which is a generic name for the antonym of 'polite'. If the concept 'rude' were part of that system, and if it were recognized as the antonym of 'polite', the statement would mean that 'sticking out your tongue' is an exemplar of 'rude'. The projector (not A) means projecting the antonym of 'A', thus making it part of the scene. On the other hand, the projector, (,not, A) means disabling 'A', so that 'A' could not participate in a wider projected scene.

When mutually exclusive concepts are joined to form new expressions, conflicts may be created in the information structure. Arbitrary statements that contain the concept 'not' may produce conflicts, because the concept 'A' and 'not A' are mutually exclusive. For example, the instruction to project ((B,is-a,A), and, (B,is-a,(not A))) is conflicting. It activates a node 'B', and declares it as an exemplar of 'A' and of 'not A', which is a conflict.

Innate exemplar-class relationships and is-a

Usually, basic atomic concepts are innately assigned as exemplars to innate class nodes. For example, all the individual point-light sensors, which cover the visual arena, are exemplars of the class 'a pixel of light'. Being exemplars of that class encodes their common property of representing a point of light. The innate sensations of hunger and thirst, for example, are exemplars of the innate class 'unpleasant state of the body'. All such innate exemplar-class relationships affect how the system parses and perceives the world. These exemplar-class relationships are encoded in the system by the weights of the connections between the exemplar nodes and the class nodes. However, the system cannot perceive connections: it can only perceive activation patterns. Is-a is the asymmetric relational concept that enables the system to perceive the existence of an exemplar-class tie between two nodes. The 'is-a' node fires when connected to an active exemplar-class pair. For example, the information that 'Rocky is a dog' is encoded in the system by a node that represents 'Rocky', a node that represents 'dog', and an exemplar-class connection between 'Rocky' and 'dog'. When 'Rocky' and 'dog' fire, the node 'is-a', which represents the relational concept 'is-a', fires, thus signaling to the rest of the system that 'Rocky' is an exemplar of 'dog'. The 'is-a' innate relational concept can also detect the relationship between acquired concepts.

Innate part-item relationships and **has-a**

Quite often, basic atomic concepts are grouped together dynamically through the part-item relationship. For example, when we hold a pencil, a large number of skin pixels in our fingers are activated. We perceive all of them as belonging to the same item. The pixels have been assigned dynamically as parts to an item. The system assigns pixels to items automatically, as situations evolve. The model represents a parts-item system by a group of inter-connected nodes. The weights of the connections from the parts to the item-node encode the conditions that if all the part-nodes are firing, the item node fires. The weights of the ties from the item-node to the parts encode the conditions that if the item-node is firing, each of its part-nodes will fire too. The **has-a** is an innate, asymmetric relational concept that enables the system to be aware of part-item relationships, the same way that the is-a relational concept enables the system to perceive the exemplar-class relationship. The relational concept 'has-a' is represented by a node that fires when its input consists of a firing part-item pair.

Sameness and perceiving objects

An object that moves across the visual field of view is perceived as one entity. In reality, different patterns of firing neurons represent a moving object at different times. The object may even look different at different distances from the observer. Internal mechanisms of information processing determine that all these patterns represent the same object. **Sameness** is a basic concept that the system uses to group patterns that occur at different times, and treat them as one entity. With experience, the basic concept of sameness is generalized and the brain can decide that two patterns that were present at far apart times are the same item, e.g. a child and an adult. Sameness is one of the most important relational concepts of the system. Through sameness, the system can treat a time sequence of varying patterns as different manifestations of the **same object**. This 'same object' is represented by an item node, whose time varying parts are the different patterns that were determined by the system to have the property of sameness.

Identical, different, and similar

When we look at twins, we say that they are identical, even though their images stimulate two different groups of light receptors in the retinas of our eyes. When we close our eyes and we hold a small item in our right hand and another identical item in our left hand, we can tell that they are identical. Again, the items have stimulated different groups of receptors in our hands. We can also determine when two entities that were present at different times are identical. The concept of being **identical** is a basic concept of the system, and it applies to information structures in various modules. Two basic relational concepts are based on the concept 'identical'. The relational concept **different**, which is its opposite, and the concept **similar**. Two information structures are **similar** to each other if corresponding parts of their structures are identical, but some of their parts are different.

Opposite and reflexive

Some innate atomic concepts that are exemplars of the same class relate to each other as **opposites**, a basic relationship that appears in many modules. Flexing a muscle and stretching it are examples of opposite basic atomic concepts of the motor module, which are recognized by the system. Pleasant and unpleasant are opposite atomic concepts of the feeling module. Some relational concepts have opposites too, e.g. 'same' and 'different'. If two asymmetric concepts are opposites of each other, they are reflexive: If the first variable of the first concept is the same as the second variable of the opposite concept, and the second variable of the first concept is the same as the first variable of the opposite, then the two concepts are the same. For example, (A,greater,B) and (B,smaller,A) are the same.

The perception of time

The flow of time is an external phenomenon, which is processed by the brain. In the model, the concept of time is treated as an information structure, which is represented by interconnected nodes. The abstract concept **time** is represented by a class node, whose exemplar nodes are **time-instances**. As time flows, the system keeps recruiting nodes to represent the passing time-instances. The rate at which the system recruits the time-instance nodes is a parameter of the system. The recruited nodes are used to organize recorded memories in chronological order. All recorded events that have happened at the same time have the node that represents that time-instance as their part. An event that has spanned over a longer period has all the corresponding time-instance nodes as its parts. Figure 4.4 illustrates the relationships between nodes that represent time concepts and nodes that record other events.

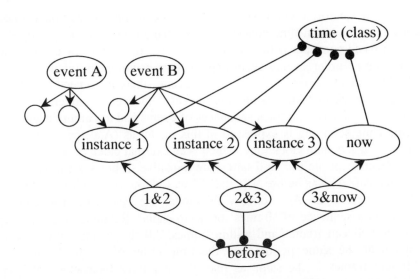

Figure 4.4: Representing time. The class node 'time' has exemplars that represent time instances. The time order of these instances is recorded by the relational concept 'before', according to the scheme shown (not all the connections are shown here). Events A and B have their part nodes (circles). In addition, event A has the node that represents time-instance 1 as its part. Event B, which has happened during the period represented by time-instance nodes 1, 2 and 3, has those nodes as its parts.

The model has basic relational concepts dealing with time, which are represented by nodes, and which have their detectors: **before** and **at the same time**. Before is an asymmetric transitive concept. If event 1 happened before event 2, they recruit a node 1&2 to represent them. This node becomes an exemplar of the class-node 'before', according to the scheme illustrated in figure 4.4.

Two recorded events that have happened at the same time will have as a part the node that represents the same time-instance. The same-time detector will fire when presented with these two events. As time progresses, a new 'now' node is recruited and becomes part of the time information structure, including the appropriate ties with the 'before' class-node.

The concepts **before** and **after** are two relational concepts that indicate the time order of two events, e.g. (A,before,B). As opposite, asymmetric, relational concepts, they are reflexive, and are members of the relational structure ((A,before,B),same,(B,after,A)), that contains the relational concept **same**. The relational time concepts 'at the same time', 'before', and 'after' are the basic concepts with which we perceive time order of events. They enable us to order events according to their occurrences relative to each other. In order to perceive time order of events, there is no need to rely on a universal clock to 'time stamp' each event. However, a universal external clock makes it easier to track sequences of events and to communicate about them. Time stamping is expressed in this model as (A,at the same time,t), where 't' is a certain clock time, which is an external clock event.

The concept 'before' and 'after' are transitive. If our system has explicit records that 'A' was before 'B', and 'B' was before 'C', we can deduce that 'A' was before 'C'. According to the model, the system records sequential events as a sequence of 'frames' or 'snap shots'. Relational time concepts operate between frames and within frames. All the events within a frame happen at the same period, and the time order of events belonging to different frames is the same as that of the frames themselves. All these relationships can be deduced by the system if they are not recorded explicitly.

Proximity

The system has internal scale by which it can compare two occurrences of the same multi-valued concept. If the two are not identical, the system can determine if they are close to each other or far from each other, according to the internal scale. For example, if we touch two objects, we can tell if their temperatures are about the same or significantly different. If we lift two objects, we can tell (based on the tension in our muscles that is needed to lift them or the pressure in our palms) if their weights is about the same or not. When we look at objects we can tell if they are close to each other or not. The sensation of elapsed time is another example of a multi-valued concept that has an internal scale. The relational, multi-valued, symmetrical concept **proximity** is a basic concept, which has different meanings in different modules. The internal scales of the various proximity concepts have default values, which may change with time and can be adjusted.

More and less, gradient

The values of some multi-valued concepts can be compared and ordered. Consequently, we can say that one sound is louder than the other, or that it feels more tiring to run uphill than to run downhill. **More** and **less** are two opposite, asymmetric, relational, and transitive concepts. If (A,more,B) and (B,more,C) then (A,more,C). Projectors of these concepts simulate situations such that the transitivity can be detected by the detectors of these concepts. When a multi-valued property of two neighboring pixels is not the same, there is a **gradient** of that property, meaning that the property changes with the position of the node in its arena. The direction of the gradient is from the pixel with the higher value to the pixel with the lower value.

Cause, if then

In addition to being able to perceive what is the time order of two events, the system can notice that whenever a certain event is present, another one always follows. This relationship is expressed by the asymmetric relational concept of **cause**. The concept of (A, cause,B) is equivalent to the concept of 'if A then B.and. A,before,B'. In the context of the model, 'if A then B' means that if A happens (exists, fires) then B happens (exists, fires). The concept of causality is fundamental to science, and a lot of effort is devoted to distinguish between causal and coincidental relationships (e.g. some specific symptoms that precede a heart attack are not its cause). The brain may need several experiences to refine the distinction between cause and sequential coincidence. Occasionally, the brain may erroneously characterize coincidental relationships between events as causal.

Repeat

As a detector, (,repeat,A)? fires when the same event happens at two different times. The concept 'repeat' consists of the more basic concepts of 'after' and 'same'. As a projector, it causes the same event to be projected at two different times. The repeated event may be a part of a more general event, which is implicitly repeated as a whole. When the projector 'repeat' acts directly or indirectly on itself, an infinite sequence of repetitions ensues, because the node 'repeat' keeps activating itself.

Combinations of temporal and other basic concepts

The basic temporal properties of any concept are the present/absent states, which are simulated by a firing/quiet node, respectively. These properties can be detected and projected by **presence** (or **at the same time**) detectors and projectors, which operate in all the modules. The basic relational concept of **starting** represents a relationship between two consecutive temporal states of the same concept. The concept was not present at the first time interval, and became present after that. Similarly, **ongoing**, and **ending** are relational temporal concepts with the obvious meanings. The relational temporal concepts of **increasing** and **decreasing** indicate temporal relationships between different values of the same multi-valued concept.

The concept of **time interval** between events is a basic relational concept. It is a class whose exemplars are time intervals between various events. These exemplars can be compared through the concept of **longer time**, which is a transitive asymmetric relational concept that is activated by pairs of 'time intervals'. The opposite concept is **shorter time**. There are some default time intervals in the system, and the relational concept (A,long,) indicates that the particular time interval 'A' is longer than the default time interval. **Short** has similar meaning. **Quick** means that the time interval between two events was short, and **slow** means that the time interval was long.

System-wide basic constructors

Constructors are represented by nodes, which are triggered by the activity of other nodes. However, unlike relational concepts, constructors' activities result in structural changes in the network. They recruit nodes to represent new concepts, establish new ties, and trim and change weights of existing ties. Each constructor has an inverse, which reverses its effects. The effects of a constructor may be long or short lasting. It all depends if and when its changes are reversed by its inverse. The notations of constructors are similar to those of relational concepts. Square brackets indicate a constructor e.g. [A,constructor,B]. The innate constructors are:

Recruit

The **recruit** constructor recruits an unassigned node, and makes it a member of an information structure. The 'recruit' constructor operates in conjunction with constructors that establish ties between nodes. A standalone node, which is not connected to any assigned node in the system, is meaningless. The constructor **dismiss** is the opposite of recruit. It disconnects all existing ties to a node, thus making it unassigned.

Connect/disconnect

Connect [A,connect-weight,B] is an asymmetrical constructor that operates on two assigned nodes of the database. It establishes a synapse of strength 'weight' from node 'A' to node 'B'. If a synapse already exists, it updates its strength to 'weight'. If 'weight' is equal to zero, the synapse from 'A' to 'B' is **disconnected**. A variant of connect is **Increase-weight**. The constructor [A,increase-weight-dw,B] increases the strength of the existing synapse from 'A' to 'B' by dw. If dw is negative, the strength is decreased.

Tie/Untie

Ties, which are bi-directional connections between nodes, are manipulated by pairs of 'connect' constructors, one in each direction. These pairs of 'connect' constructors constitute the four basic **tie** constructors, which form the corresponding tie from node 'A' to node 'B': [A,tie-part-to-item,B], [A,tie-itemi-to-part,B], [A,tie-exemplar-to-class,B], [A,tie-class-to-exemplar,B]. The tie constructor operates on a single pair. When an item-node is recruited to represent a group of part-nodes, it is necessary to record the relationship of the group as a whole to its item node. If the sum of all the weights from the part-nodes to the item is exactly one, all the parts have to fire in order to activate the item-node. That can be accomplished by the **normalize** constructor. The constructor [A,normalize-sum,B] normalizes the weights from a group of parts 'A' to their item-node 'B' so that the sum of their weights is 'sum'. 'Sum' may be any number. **Untie** is the operation in which a bi-directional tie is disconnected.

Switch

Switch is a constructor that unties one node from a second node, and then ties a third node to the second node, with the same type of tie. It is a combination of the basic constructors 'tie' and 'untie', but because of its prevalence, it could be considered a basic concept. The notation [A,B,switch,C] indicates that 'A' is untied from 'B', and then 'C' is tied to 'B' with the same tie that existed between 'A' and 'B'.

Modulate

A **modulate** constructor multiplies all the current outgoing weights in a bundle by the same modulation factor. There are four modulate constructors, for the four bundle groups: [A,modulate-part-item,factor], [A,modulate-item-part,factor],   [A,modulate-exemplar-class,factor],   [A,modulate-class-exemplar,factor]. When 'factor' is zero, the bundle is disabled. When 'factor' is negative, the bundle is reset to its default value.

Explicate/implicate

Concepts are connected to each other by exemplar-class and by part-item connections. Since these connections are transitive, the presence of a node in a situation implies that all its parts and all its classes could also be present. However, in reality, that does not always happen. Only some of the parts and classes of an active node are active too. Occasionally, the system needs to activate some dormant class and part nodes of an active node, so that more details about a situation at hand become available. The constructor **explicate** is used for that purpose. [,explicate,A] activates all the part nodes and class nodes that are directly connected to node 'A'. It may accomplish this goal by modulating the appropriate bundles, if their default multiplication factors were set at less than one. The inverse concept of explicate is **implicate**. It reduces the number of active class and part nodes of an active node by reducing the appropriate modulation factors.

Clone

Cloning is an operation that generates a replica of a given information structure. The constructor [A,clone,B] creates an information structure 'B', which has the same internal and external connections as information structure 'A'.

Module-specific relational concepts

Concept structures in the visual module

The visual arena consists of pixels with their pixel's-clusters. The color of a pixel and the intensity of that color are multi-valued atomic concepts represented by two nodes in each pixel's-cluster, as shown in figure 4.1. System-wide relational concepts act with these visual atomic concepts and form joint concepts. For example, the basic relational concept 'increase' together with 'color intensity' constitute the concept of 'increase of color intensity', which is represented by its own node in the corresponding pixel array. Relational temporal concepts that are based on the system-wide 'presence' and 'absence' concepts can describe various temporal sequences of pixel's illumination e.g. flickering. Nodes that represent such joint concepts are added to the pixel's-clusters. In addition to such joint concepts, there are relational concepts that are purely visual. These relational concepts describe certain spatial and temporal relationships between patterns of active pixels of the visual module.

Retinal and world coordinate systems: There are many similarities between the eye and the camera. Both have a lens, which receives rays of light from external objects. The lens is controlled by a focusing mechanism, which ensures that a sharp image of the observed object is projected onto a surface behind the lens. In the camera, this surface is the film, which is covered by photosensitive material. In the eye, this surface is the retina, which is covered by photoreceptors. If we turn the camera, while it is still 'looking' at the object, the image will rotate on the film. That is how we sometimes fit a tall object into the picture. We turn the camera so that its long side lies parallel to the tall object. Similarly, if we turn our head from the upright position towards one shoulder, the projected image will rotate on the retina. However, when we look at an object while turning our head towards the shoulder, the object seems to stay put. It does not rotate. The brain keeps a stable image of the rotating retinal image. It can be said that while the mesh of pixels in the retina form a retinal coordinate system, the brain perceives the world through another coordinate system, which will be called **the world coordinate system**. The transformation of images from the retinal coordinate system to the world coordinate system is mediated by the vestibular system. This transformation does not depend on the individual viewed object. Whatever is displayed in the retinal coordinate system is transformed to the world coordinate system, which is aligned with respect to the ubiquitous gravitational field. Consequently, the world coordinate system has fixed **top** and **bottom**, and **up** and **down directions**. We know that the ceiling is above us and the floor is bellow irrespective of the orientation of our head. The basic concept **horizontal** is also defined relative to up and down in the world coordinate system. The basic relational concepts **in front of me, behind me, to my left, to my right**, and their refinements refer to situations in the retinal coordinate system. For example, (an-object ,in-front-of, me) means an object whose image is at the center of the retina when my head is in normal position; (an-object,to-the-left-of,me) means that when I turn my head to the left, the image of the object will be at the center of the retina. The concepts of spatial relationships between two objects, such as

above, below, to the side, in front, behind, etc., and their refinements are basic relational concepts of the visual module. The arena of the visual module consists of the two inter-related world and retinal coordinate systems. The various concepts can be represented in the appropriate coordinate system, as applicable.

Although the retina is a two-dimensional surface, we perceive through it the three dimensional world. This is accomplished in part due to having two eyes that see the same object from two angles, and in part due to learning from experience. We can grasp the three dimensional contents of a scene from its two dimensional picture. The model presented here does not specify the details of the mechanisms used by the brain to process two-dimensional information and create from it three-dimensional perceptions. It assumes that the detectors that detect three-dimensional concepts do so from the two dimensional images in the visual arena, and that the projectors of three-dimensional concepts project the appropriate two-dimensional images onto the visual arena.

Innate grouping: The visual module **group**s active pixels that have similar features into items. Imagine a piece of white paper on which two stripes, one red and one green, have been painted. It takes almost no time for an observer to conclude that there are two objects, a red one and a green one, on the paper. The brain has grouped all the red pixels into one object, and all the greens into another. Nodes in inner layers of the module are recruited to represent such items, whose parts are firing pixels in the input layer. Grouping can be based on a variety of common active features of pixels. For example, the flickering lights on a Christmas tree are perceived as parts of one entity, in addition to being recognized individually. Recruited nodes that represent patterns of the input layer act, in turn, as pixels to nodes deeper in the module, and so on for several levels.

An **edge** in the visual field is a relational innate concept. The system is wired to detect abrupt spatial changes of color, intensity of color, and other properties that are represented by nodes of pixel's-clusters. Adjacent pixels in which an abrupt change of a feature occurs, are grouped by the system to form an edge. Edges are sometimes used by the system to parse a scene into smaller patterns whose pixels are grouped to form items.

Grouping is a dynamic process, and its outcome depends on the actual objects, which are present in the field of view. However, some grouped items occur frequently in our environment, and they form classes of relational concepts in their own right, e.g. **line, straight line, closed line**

open line, **end of line**, **surface**, **plane**, **corner**, etc. These are class concepts, and a group of points that satisfy certain relational conditions becomes an item, which is an exemplar of the corresponding class. More complex **geometrical objects**, such as squares or pyramids, are relational concepts that are built from the more basic geometrical concepts.

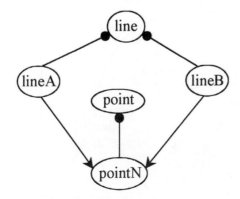

Figure 4.5: Representing the information that lineA and lineB intersect.

Topological relationships: The basic relational concepts between two open lines: **strange to each other** and **intersect** are easily expresses by more fundamental concepts. For example, the concept **intersect**: (lineA, intersect,lineB) can be expressed as: There is a point 'pointN' that belongs to 'lineA' and to 'lineB'. In the language of the model this is expressed as: ((lineA, is_a,line),and,(lineB,is_a,line), and,(pointN,is_a,point), and, (lineA,has_a,pointN), and,(lineB,has_a,pointN),and,(lineA,different,lineB)). The information structure that represents this situation in shown in figure 4.5.

Figure 4.6 shows the schematics of an intersection detector. The detector is continuously observing pixels in a region of the visual arena, and it fires when it detects intersecting lines. It contains two line detectors, a point detector, two 'has-a' detectors, and a difference detector. When the appropriate input enters the circuitry of the intersection detector, each of the constituting detectors fires, causing the intersection detector to fire. This indicates the presence of an intersection. The actual intersection point is the input of the point detector.

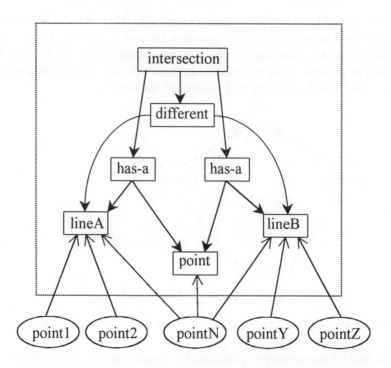

Figure 4.6: A structure of detectors that detects intersections of two lines (inside dotted square). The detectors are marked by squares. LineA and lineB are two line detectors, and 'point' is a point detector that accepts only one variable. When all the parts of an item-detector fire, the item-detector fires.

In retrieval mode, nodes that represent a cue are activated in the circuitry of the detector. A solution is obtained when other nodes join the cue and activate the detector. For example, if a line that intersect a given line has to be found, the points of the given line, say point1, point2, and pointN, are activated as the cue. A group of nodes that would cause the intersection detector to fire, such as pointY and pointZ, define a solution.

In projection mode, a set of default pixels, which form intersecting lines, are activated in the visual arena.

Closed lines in a plane divide the plane into two regions. Any point in the plane, which is not a part of the line, satisfies one of the relational concepts: **inside the line** or **outside the line.** Similarly, closed surfaces divide the space into two regions: **inside the surface** and **outside the surface**. The brain applies the concepts of inside and outside also to open (concave) geometrical shapes. It does it by treating the **gap** too as a part of the shape. This is illustrated in figure 4.7:

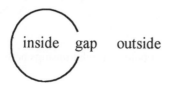

Figure 4.7 The concepts of inside and outside of an open curve.

The topological relationships between two closed lines in a plane (or closed surfaces in space) are basic relational concepts of the visual module. These include the symmetric relationships of **strange to each other, touch from the outside, intersect** (part inside, part outside), and **overlap**; and the asymmetrical relational concepts **touch from the inside** and **contain**, as illustrated in figure 4.8:

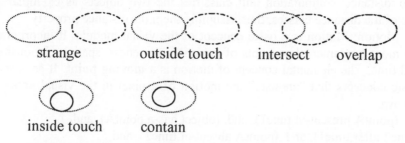

Figure 4.8: Concepts of topological relationships for closed shapes.

These concepts can be constructed with the fundamental concepts of: point, line, inside, outside, is-a, has-a, all, and there-is. They can be extended to relationships between open shapes. Figure 4.9 illustrates the relationships 'contain', 'intersect', and 'strange' when open shapes are involved:

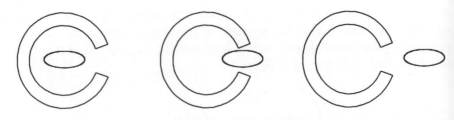

Figure 4.9: Concepts of topological relationships between open shapes.

Distance: The concept of **distance** between two objects in the field of view is the visual module's realization of the general concept of proximity. It is an ordered concept that operates on topologically strange objects. It has grades from very close to very far. Depending on the situation, the brain may use various mechanisms to determine the distance between two objects. Scientifically, distance can be expressed by numbers. However, the brain uses subjective methods, which sometimes do not conform to the scientific determination. In the model, the distance detector is a computation unit whose inputs are the images of the objects as represented in the visual arena. The 'distance' computation unit classifies the two objects as exemplars of one of the distance classes, thus assigning them the distance property.

Motion: Motion is a basic concept of the visual module. It incorporates the more fundamental concepts of grouping, sameness, spatial relationships, and time. The elemental concept of motion is a **moving point**. It consists of basic concepts that "animate" the motion of a pixel in the visual arena, as follows:

(pointA,present-at,time1), and, (object,has-a,pointA), and,
(time2,after,time1), and ,(pointA,absent-at,time2), and,
(pointB,different,pointA), and ,(pointB,present-at,time2), and, (object,has-a,pointB).

Moving points are assembled by the brain into objects that have time-dependent and time-independent properties. The brain is able to distinguish between the two broad categories of **moving object**s and objects that undergo shape change

A moving object creates in the visual arena patterns of firing pixels that change with time. Pixels that fire concurrently are grouped into 'snapshots'. Each of the snapshots, in its turn, becomes a temporary part of a fixed item-node that represents the moving object. That item-node may have also fixed relationships with other nodes in the system. For example, a moving car is represented by a fixed node 'a moving car'. The images of the car in the visual arena change with time (a sequence of snapshots), and constitute time-varying parts of the node 'a moving car'. These snapshots consist of pixels, which correspond to the car's position and shape, and of their pixel's-clusters, which describe other pixel properties, such as color. In addition, if the car is a fire-truck, the node 'a moving car' is an exemplar of the class-node 'fire-truck'. That exemplar-class relation does not depend on time. Because of it, the node 'a moving car' inherits all the properties of a fire-truck e.g. the typical siren sound, a record of which is stored in the auditory module. Every moving object that the system perceives is represented in such a way.

There are many motion concepts that moving objects may have. These are expressed as ties between the 'moving object' node and nodes that represent those concepts. For example, **move to the right** and **move to the left** are two basic motion concepts. If car A moves to the right, and car B moves to the left, car A is an exemplar of 'objects moving to the right' and car B is an exemplar of 'objects moving to the left'.

The concept '**moving object**' is an information structure that consists of hierarchies of classes and exemplars. The following is a list of some of those concepts: object moves from point A to point B; object moves in direction D; object moves at speed S; object spinning at frequency F around X; concepts that involve the self such as I move from point A to point B; I move in direction D; I move at speed S; I spin at frequency F around X, where A and B indicate pixels. The variables of these concepts are themselves hierarchies of concepts: the symbol D indicates one of the available directional concepts such as to the left, upwards, away, ahead, etc. A given direction is a basic concept that incorporates the more fundamental concepts of straight line and ordered scanning of a group of points (to be discussed soon). The symbol S indicates the speed of the motion. We can express speed by exact numerical values e.g. miles per hour. However, the instinctive perception of speed is different. **Speed** is an ordered non-numerical concept. We can describe in broad terms how fast an object is moving, and that one object is moving faster than another. Our perception is not always scientifically correct. For example, we may perceive the speed of a racecar greater than that of the sun in the sky. The symbol F indicates how fast the object is spinning, and around which imaginary axis X. Similar to S, F can be expressed by numbers, but the system treats it as a non-numerical ordered concept. The system can attribute these motion concepts to objects in the field of view and to the self. Different mechanisms are involved in these two kinds of attribution. They are supported by the model but their details are beyond its scope.

More complex motion patterns can be expressed as sequences of segments of these elemental motions. Sometimes, words describe in a concise way combinations of more fundamental concepts. For example, **oscillate** means moving in one direction, reaching a point, moving in the opposite direction, reaching another point, moving in the first direction, etc.

Changing shape is another information structure that consists of hierarchies of concepts. Some of the included concepts are: **contracting, expanding, stretching, squeezing, shearing, twisting, bending, straightening, bulging, denting,** etc. All these basic concepts can be decomposed into the more fundamental concepts that have already been mentioned above. For example, (,contract,A) may be expressed as: (time2,after,time1),and ,(A,present-at, time1),and ,(A,absent-at,time2),and ,(B,absent at,time1),and ,(B,present-at,time2), and, (A,contain,B),and ,(A,same,B).

Kinetic relationships between objects. There are relational concepts that characterize two objects that move in the field of view. They include: **approaching, moving away, colliding, one hit the other, bouncing, moving together, moving in parallel, spinning around each other, entering, penetrating, engulfing, passing through, exiting, filling, emptying,** and so on. These concepts are combinations of the more fundamental concepts mentioned above. For example (A,enter,B) may be expressed as: (time2,after,time1),and ,(time3,after,time2),and ,(B,has-a,gap),and ,(B,has-a,inside),and ,((A,outside,B),at,time1),and ,((A,move-to,gap),at, time2),and ,((A,move to,inside),at, time3).

Divide, combine: Divide is a basic relational concept of the form (A,divide,**B**). It pertains to the situation in which one item divides into a group of items. Each of the resulting items has its own item node. The fundamental relational concept 'divide' assumes that no motion or change of shape are involved in the division. Every pixel that belonged to 'A' will belong to one of the concepts of '**B**', and will carry with it its pixel's-clusters properties that do not change with the division. Pixel's-cluster properties that may change in division are 'being on the edge', 'not being on an edge', and the likes. Relationships between A and its classes are voided. For example, the pieces of a broken chair have wood properties. However, not all edge properties of the original chair pixels prevail, and the broken pieces do not belong to the class 'chair'. After the fundamental division, properties of items of '**B**' are updated according to the situation. 'Divide' can be expressed by more fundamental relational-concepts. For example, a situation in which (l,m,n,o,and p) are parts of 'A', and 'A' divides into 'C'=(l,m,n) and 'D'=(o,p) can be expressed as: (time2,after,time1), and, ((A,untie,*l,m,n,o,p*),at,time1),and ,(((,recruit,C),and ,(,recruit,D),and.(C,tie-item-parts,*l,m,n*),and,(D,tie- item-parts,*o,p*),at,time2).

Combine is the inverse of 'divide'. The following will reverse the last 'divide':
(time2,after,time1),and ,((D,untie,*o,p*),and ,(C,untie,*l,m,n*),at,time1),and ,(((,recruit,A),and ,(A,tie item parts,*l,m,n,o,p*),at,time2).

The concepts divide and combine are elements in a variety of other concepts, which are derived by adding more details about the variables 'A' and 'B'. For example, **break, split, cut, chop, dice, explode, multiply, spray, mix, dissolve, fuse,** etc.

Object dependent relational concepts: Many concepts that have their own words describe situations in which specific objects participate in the basic relational-concepts mentioned above. For example: **fly** = move inside air; **high** = far above ground; **soar** = fly high; **sink** = move down in water; **dive** = move down in air, then penetrate water, then sink. '**A**' **is connected to** '**B**' = 'A' and 'B' are touching from outside and their points of contact are the same at different times.

A large group of concepts consists of a time-dependent visual component and an object that causes the visual changes. For example, **to dress** = cause an item to contain part of a human so that that part touches-from-inside the clothing item. **Object** '**A**' **pushes object** '**B**' = Object 'A' is touching from outside object 'B', and object 'A' causes object 'B' to move away from 'A'.

Concept structures in the auditory module

The atomic concepts of the auditory module are pitch, tone-quality, and tone-intensity. Pitch and tone-intensity have well-established physical and physiological correlates. Sound waves that reach the ear cause vibrations that propagate in the basilar membrane. When the sound wave is sinusoidal, those propagating vibrations peak at one point on the membrane. The location of the peak depends on the frequency of the sound wave that has caused it. The higher the frequency of the sound wave, the closer the peak of the vibrating membrane to the base of the membrane. The height of the peak depends on the intensity of the sound wave. The greater the sound intensity, the higher the peak of the membrane. Hair cells, which act as sensing auditory pixels, pick up the corresponding displacements of the membrane, and relay that information to the neural network. However, there is no one to one correspondence between sound frequencies and their activated hair pixels. A hair cell will usually respond in different amounts to different frequencies.

In general, sounds are not pure sinusoidal waves. Rather, they consist of superposition of pure sinusoidal waves of various frequencies, intensities, and duration. The tone-quality of a certain pitch is due to superposition of harmonics of the fundamental pitch frequency. (Harmonics are frequencies that are multiples of the fundamental pitch frequency.) The brain cannot separate the individual harmonics that make up a given tone-quality. This is similar to the situation in the visual module, where the brain cannot separate the intensities of the red, blue, and green components that make up the perceived color of a certain visual pixel.

Since humans can discern pitch, tone-quality, and tone intensity, these may serve as the basic auditory concepts of the model. The auditory pixels of the model are characterized by their pitch (frequency). The pixel's-clusters contain nodes that represent the features of tone-quality and tone intensity. At any given time, several tone-quality nodes, with their intensity nodes, may be active. This simulates situations such as listening to a duet, when we can recognize the pitch and intensity of the sounds emitted by each of the singers. The schematic structure of an auditory pixel's-cluster was shown in figure 4.2

Different individuals have different levels of musical acuity. For example, a good conductor can notice what each instrument of the orchestra is playing, while an ordinary listener may be able to discern only a few instruments. The implication is that the extent of the details in the auditory network, as modeled in figure 4.2, depends on the individual.

The relational concept **same pitch** means that two tones, which may differ in their tone-quality, have the same fundamental pitch, and are exemplars of the same pitch node. The relational concept **same tone-quality** means that two tones have the same spectrum of harmonics. Tone-quality distinguishes between sources of different nature, such as different musical instruments. It is also one of the characterizing features of the voices of different human speakers. Detectors of 'same tone-quality' may be important elements in parsing an auditory scene according to the sources of its sounds. The relational concept **same sound pattern** is an extension of the concept 'same tone-quality'. It pertains to general frequency and temporal patterns that characterize sound sources. For example, we can listen to one person over the background of other voices and sounds, based on the particular pattern of auditory features of that voice. The first stages of this kind of information processing takes place in a circuitry like figure 4.2

Pitch and tone-intensity are ordered concepts. The relational concepts **higher pitch** and **louder sound** pertain to comparisons of atomic auditory concepts. The atomic properties that feed these relational concepts are represented by nodes that belong to the pixel's-clusters in figure 4.2.

When playing a familiar tune on a piano, one can start it at any key of the keyboard (this is called transposition). The actual sound waves in the air of two transposed versions of the same tune will be different from each other. Still, a listener would identify the played tune whether it started with a do, a sol, or any other note. That is an indication that the auditory module has some innate relational concepts that facilitate such perceptions.

The fundamental frequencies of the notes of the chromatic musical scale (do, do-sharp, re, re-sharp, mi, fa, etc.) have an interesting property. The ratio between the frequencies of any two consecutive notes is almost the same. That ratio is equal to 1.059 for any two consecutive notes of the chromatic scale. For example, the ratio between the frequencies of fa and mi is 1.059, the same as the ratio between the frequencies of do-sharp and do. The ratio between the frequencies of any two notes can be expresses as 1.059 to the power of a positive or negative integer (1.059^n, where n is a positive or negative integer). When n=12, the frequency ratio between the two notes is 2:1, which corresponds to one octave. The **frequency-ratio** between the frequencies represented by two pitch nodes is a basic relational concept of the auditory module. Prevalent frequency-ratios are represented by their own nodes. A frequency-ratio detector will fire when the frequency ratio between its first and second input nodes matches its specific value. A memory record of a tune can be expressed as a sequence of the frequency-ratios of its notes. Two renditions of the same tune, which are different only by their starting note, will have the same sequence of frequency-ratio values. After specifying the starting note, frequency-ratio projectors can unfold and playback the entire tune.

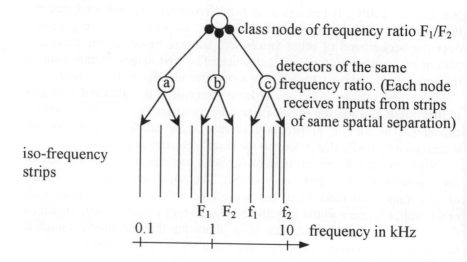

class node of frequency ratio F_1/F_2

detectors of the same frequency ratio. (Each node receives inputs from strips of same spatial separation)

iso-frequency strips

F_1 F_2 f_1 f_2

0.1   1   10   frequency in kHz

Figure 4.10: Detecting frequency ratios in the auditory module. Iso-frequency strips (pixel's-clusters of pitch nodes) are separated proportionally to the logarithm of their frequencies (bottom scale). They are observed by similar detectors. Detectors b and c detect the same frequency ratio $F_1/F_2=f_1/f_2$.

The details of the mechanisms that the brain uses to detect frequency ratios are beyond the scope of this model. The following is one possible biological realization of that process, which is compatible with the general principles of the model, and thus it could be incorporated in it. This example illustrates how factors other than connectivity between neurons may play a role in feature detection. There are some indications that frequency-ratio nodes are feasible in biological systems. Areas of the auditory cortex of the dog are organized tonotopically: Iso-frequency strips, which are reminiscent of the columns in the primary visual cortex, have been identified and mapped in the auditory cortex of the dog (Tunturi, 1952). The distances between strips seem to be proportional to the logarithm of their frequencies (figure 4.10). Consider now four strips, representing the frequencies F_1, F_2, f_1, and f_2. The distance between cortical strips F_1 and F_2 is the same as the distance between f_1 and f_2. Because of the logarithmic scale (bottom of figure 4.8) this means that log F_1-log F_2 = log f_1- log f_2, which means that $F_1/F_2=f_1/f_2$. These strips are being observed by detectors of similar structures. Detector b fires when pixels F_1 and F_2 fire, and detector c fires when pixels f_1 and f_2 fire. In other words, the detectors detect the frequency ratio $F_1/F_2=f_1/f_2$. Logarithmic slide-rulers are based on the same principle. Detectors b and c are exemplars of the class 'frequency ratio of F_1/F_2'.

The auditory module generates and maintains records of various sounds that the system has encountered. It has detectors, and it keeps records of various voices and of sounds of phonemes and words, which are expressed as temporal patterns of atomic and relational concepts that were described above.

The motor module

The atomic concepts of the motor module are nodes that send activation instructions to individual motor units. These nodes are the pixels of the motor module, and they operate as output-only pixels. The nodes of their pixel's-clusters represent various intensities of contraction. The instructions to contract are multi-valued, and they encode the intensity of the contraction of the muscle unit. They can be formulated as (,contract-intensity, X), where **contract-intensity** indicates the intensity of the contraction of motor unit X. When 'intensity' is zero the muscle unit is completely relaxed, and when 'intensity' is negative the muscle is inhibited. Basic concepts of the motor module are temporal patterns of these atomic instructions. They involve coordinated activation of groups of motor units. These basic concepts can be detected and projected like any other basic concepts of other modules. The motor module has action plans, which involve basic motor concepts and feedback from other modules, such as the posture module and other sensory modules.

An important relational concept, which is typical to the motor unit, is **reverse operation**. There are two kinds of reverse operations, depending on the involved muscle units. If the muscle unit has an antagonist unit, such as the triceps and the biceps, a reverse operation will affect both units. It will relax the currently contracted unit and contract its currently relaxed or stretched antagonist unit. If the affected unit does not have an antagonist unit, a reverse instruction will relax a contracted unit, and will contract a relaxed unit. The system organizes its concepts such that it can detect, project, record, and retrieve reverse operations. Pairs of reverse operations are exemplars of the class of mutually exclusive concepts.

The relational concept 'reverse operation' applies also to temporal patterns of basic operations. It reverses the temporal order of the basic operations and replaces each individual operation by its reverse. For example, when we reach with our hand and grasp a hot object, the reverse operation will first open our fingers by activating the antagonist hand muscles, and then pull back our hand by activating the antagonist arm and shoulder muscles.

The central module

In addition to being an association module to all other modules, the central module is responsible for executing and recording some specialized activities.

Thinking concepts. One of the activities of the central module is thinking. In thinking, the system tries to retrieve an existing memory record, or to synthesize a novel information entity, so that it conforms to a specified query or a problem. Those conformity requirements can vary in their complexity. In their most simple cases–free associations–the only requirement is that the query and the outcome of the process are associated to each other. The specifics of the association are not prescribed. In more complex thinking, the specifics of these relationships may become very elaborate. A thinking problem, in general, has two component: the given and the constraints. The given is a data entity that is completely known. The constraints specify the relationships that have to exist between the given and the outcome of the thinking process–the solution. The constraints have some variable slots, which have to be filled by elements of the solution. The given, the constraints, and the solution are expressed by concepts, atomic and relational, which are connected to each other by the four basic relationships and their negations.

In searching for a solution, the system goes through memory records that seem to be the most relevant to the given problem. A search may uncover a complete solution or a partial one. After appraising the retrieved information, the system decides whether to end the process, or to continue and zoom-in on a more complete and detailed solution. All those phases of a thinking process are states of the central module. They are concepts, and they are represented by nodes.

Quite often, a problem will have implied constraints in addition to the explicit ones. In the search process, implied constrained are satisfied automatically. The system will send notification signals only when implied constraints are violated. The system seeks actively only solutions to the explicit constraints. For example, in chess, the problem is what moves to make in order to capture the opponent's king. Normally, the player's thoughts would concentrate on the chess pieces, and would not involve plans to confuse the opponent by a sneaky punch. That would violate the implied constraints of the problem at hand.

Thinking processes may involve sub-processes and plans, which are executed consciously and subconsciously, much like processes in the motor module. Thinking processes, sub-processes, and plans are basic concepts that are represented by nodes. The item node **thinking** has part nodes: **problem** and **solution**. The node 'problem' has **given** and **constraints** as its parts. All these are also class nodes, whose exemplars are actual thinking events and their actual components. The constructor **solve** [problem,solve-plan,solution] substitutes the actual problem into an actual thinking plan, and generates a solution. It contains sub-constructors that **evaluate the match** between the solution and the problem. The latter are relational constructors that classify (i.e. declares as exemplar of a class) which **constraint is satisfied**, which **constraint is not addressed**, which **constraint is erroneously answered**, and which **constraint is conflicting** which part of the solution. The constructor **partial problem** assembles unsatisfied parts of the problem, and defines them as a sub-problem for the constructor 'solve'. The solution to a problem can be also classified as **novel** or **familiar**. These classifications will determine how the solution should be recorded, if at all.

Scan: Scanning is an operation that is frequently used in thinking processes. Scan is a class concept that has four exemplars of obvious meanings: **scan parts, scan items, scan exemplars,** and **scan classes.** As a projector, **scan-parts** activates the parts of an item one at a time. At the end of a scan-parts projection, each of the parts of an item has been activated exactly once. Switching from one part to its next may be triggered by the activated part, or by an external event. For example, when asked to say the names of the past presidents of the country, we recall one name and say it. Saying a name triggers the recall of the next name, and so on, until the recall request triggers the response 'no more names to recall'

Two concepts, 'all' and 'there-is', are often appear in the formulation of problems. The concept **all** contains the concepts 'scan' and 'and'. It indicates that each of the scanned concepts possesses a common property. For example, it rained all week means that it rained on Sunday, and it rained on Monday, ..., and it rained on Saturday.

The concept **there-is,** when acting as an information detector, indicates that a certain cue is already represented in the system by a node. When it acts as a projector, it recruits a node, if necessary, to represent a concept that is defined by its relationships with other concepts.

These are some of the concepts that are related to thinking processes. Such concepts can be assembled in many ways, according to the specific needs of the thinking operation. Various thinking operations, which contain these concepts as elements, will be discussed in the next chapters.

Concepts involving the self

Self and outsiders

The innate system contains a group of interconnected nodes capable of sensing the body and the environment, controlling the activities of the body, and evaluating the available information. This group of nodes and their connections constitute the **innate self** of the system. Imagine that the innate system could talk. When the system would say "I see something", that would mean that a pattern of sensory nodes in the visual module are firing. The statement "I eat" would correspond to a spatio-temporal firing pattern of motor and sensory-taste nodes, which are involved in the eating process. Statements such as "I am afraid" or "I think" would correlate with firing patterns that are characteristic to these states and processes, and so on.

With time, experiences enhance and expand the innate self and create the mature self. The mature self includes concepts that are the outcomes of experiences involving the innate self and its environment. For example, consider the innate concept 'finger'. It is represented by a group of nodes that correspond to pixels of the finger. Some of those pixels can sense the mechanical state of the finger's muscles. Others sense external stimuli that act on the finger, such as pressure. Nodes that represent motor instructions that activate the finger also belong to the innate concept 'finger'. Through a variety of experiences, a baby's system develops the mature concept of a finger. First, the system uncovers and represents new relationships between the innate concepts. For example, if the nodes that activate the muscles of the finger and the nodes that sense the status of those muscles were not innately associated, they would become associated due to repeated experiences. The cause-effect relationship between the instruction to activate a muscle and its actual contraction would be encoded in the network. The baby's system would then have the information to say "I move my finger". In a similar way, the system would associate external stimuli with the information-structure of the self. For example, the visual pattern of the finger, as captured by the sensors of the visual module, becomes part of the data structure of the baby's own self.

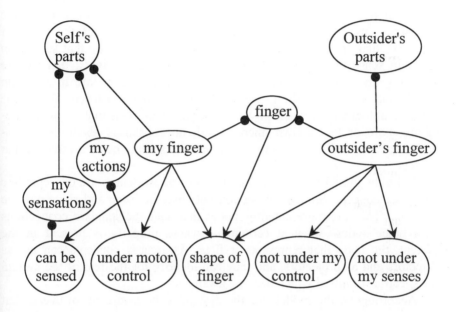

Figure 4.11: Example of relationships between 'self' and 'outsider' concepts.

The innate system contains also nodes that represent external entities. These external concepts are acquired through external sensory modules such as visual, auditory, and olfactory. The system learns to recognize these entities, which can be called **'outsiders'**, as not belonging to the self. At a certain age, children can easily distinguish between their own fingers and fingers of others. Nodes that represent outsiders and the self's nodes can activate each other, thus representing interactions between the self and the outsiders.

In the model, there are two important concept nodes–the 'self's parts' and the 'outsiders' parts'– to which many other concepts are related. All the concepts that belong to the self are exemplars of the 'self's parts' node, and all the concepts that belong to outsiders are exemplars of the 'outsiders' parts' node. Figure 4.11 illustrate typical relationships between concepts in such circuitries.

Self awareness

Self-awareness is one of the fundamental properties that humans have. We have the sensation of our presence, and we are aware of the kinds of processes that are taking place in our system. We are aware that sensors in our skin sense the air around us, that our eyes sense sights, that we are breathing, that we are thinking about something, that we are in a certain mood, and so on. In short, we are aware of our existence. While the anatomical loci and the basic physiology of the sensations that we are aware-of are more or less known, there is still no consensus about the neuro-biological loci and mechanisms of the various sensations of awareness that we feel.

From the model's perspective, sensations of awareness are concepts like any other concept. Some of these concepts may be basic and some may be acquired. They are represented by nodes that have the standard connections with other nodes. When a certain awareness property is present in the system, the node that represents it fires. Awareness concepts can act as detectors and as projectors, and they can identify for the rest of the system the specific stimuli of which they are aware.

According to the model, for the system to be aware of an event, that event has to trigger an awareness detector. Awareness detectors can thus be viewed as a distinct group of nodes that have connections with all the other nodes that the system can become aware-of.

A question comes up then about the awareness nodes themselves. Are there nodes that are aware-of other awareness nodes, and if so, how many "generations" of "aware-of-aware-of" should the system support? Although the model can provide cascades of awareness detectors, the real question is how many levels of such generation-detectors does the brain employ? It is suggested here that the system needs hardware for detecting just one generation of aware-of relationships. These detectors could be used in iterative way to represent any number of generations of aware-of relationships. To illustrate the iteration process, consider the following example. We are breathing, and we are aware that we are breathing. The act of 'breathing' is represented by a firing node (figure 4.12). The firing of this node triggers the 'activity awareness' detector, whose firing causes 'breathing' to become an exemplar of 'aware-of activities'. The two nodes 'breathing' and 'aware-of activities' can recruit a node to represent the event 'aware of breathing'. This is the representation of the first generation of awareness. The firing of the node 'aware of breathing' triggers a thought-awareness detector. The latter makes the node 'aware of breathing' belong to the class whose exemplars are thoughts that the system is aware-of. The nodes 'aware of breathing' and aware-of thoughts' recruit a node to represent them. From now on, all the generations of 'aware-of-aware-of...breathing' are detected by the same 'thought-awareness' detector, and become exemplars of the class 'aware-of thoughts' (thoughts that the system is aware-of), as illustrated in figure 4.12.

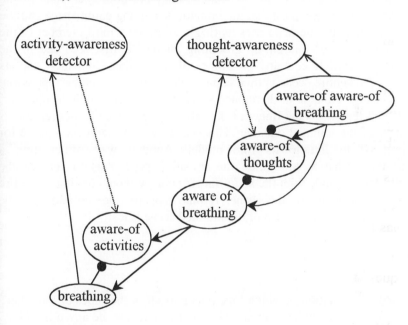

Figure 4.12: Representing "generations" of awareness of an event (breathing). The event (breathing) activates awareness detector (thin arrow), which associated the event with an awareness class (dotted arrow). The new concept (aware of breathing) is then detected by the thought-awareness detector, and the second-generation awareness concept is formed. All the following awareness-generations would be exemplars of the class 'aware-of thoughts'.

Imitate

Imitation is a widespread process used by higher level animals. The neural correlates of that process are not known, but it is reasonable to assume that the imitator constructs and uses an information structure that encodes the similarity between the activities of the imitated and corresponding activities of the self. The activities of the imitated are represented in the 'outsiders' information sub-structure of the imitator. For an imitation to be possible, there must be an association between nodes of the self and nodes that represent the imitated outsider. Figure 4.9 can serve as an example of such an association, as represented by the model. The concepts 'finger of the self' and 'finger of an outsider' are associated. They are both exemplars of the class-node 'finger'. Suppose that the imitator is a young chimpanzee and the imitated is an adult one, who uses its finger to groom a third member of the group. The scene of one chimp grooming another is first recorded in the imitator's system. It contains the finger of the imitated outsider, and its activities. This entire scene is then copied, using the basic 'clone' operation. Then, a change is made in the cloned structure, using the 'switch' operator. A node that represents the finger of the self replaces the node that represents the finger of the imitated outsider. This scene can now serve as a guide for the imitator to imitate its role model. Another way of creating a representation that would guide the imitation process is to replace the outsider's finger node with the self's finger node, without copying the entire information structure of the scene. If that happens, the imitation can be carried out, but the full record of the imitated scene is lost.

Empathize

Empathy is a situation in which 'one puts himself in the shoes of the other'. The other may be another human being, but it may also be any other entity such as a tree, a planet, or a nation, etc. Empathy has some similarities to imitation, but the main difference is that empathy must involve feelings. The model can handle empathizing by relying on the concepts 'self' and 'outsiders', and basic constructors such as 'clone' and 'switch'. First, nodes of an outsider are matched with corresponding nodes of the self. For example, when empathizing with another human, nodes that represent parts of that outsider, such as stomach, are first matched with nodes that represent the same parts of the self. When empathizing with a tree, branches of the tree may be matched with hands. Then, information structures of the self, which are connected to the matched nodes of the self, are connected also to the corresponding nodes of the outsider. When 'stomach' is the match, self's nodes that are associated with 'stomach' (e.g. nodes that represent hunger or stomach pain) are connected in a similar way to the nodes that represent the stomach of the outsider. When the match is between hands and branches, pain of the hands can be attributed also to the branches. Through such arrangements, the self can empathize with outsiders. Concepts and information structures that the self uses to analyze and describe its experiences are now used to analyze and describe experiences of the outsider. However, the combinations of concepts that the self employs to empathize with an outsider are determined by the self, and they may be different from those used by the self for dealing with its own situations. For example, the feelings that hypocrites apply to behaviors of others are different from what they apply to their own deeds.

The system can use the self's structure to empathize in different ways with different outsiders. It assigns an appropriate empathy structure to the appropriate individual. The basic relational concept (X,empathize-structure,Y) describes these processes. X stands for the empathizing entity and Y stands for the empathized. X and Y can be the self or an outsider. Empathize-structure defines the information structure used in the particular empathy process. For example, the relational concept (X,loves,Y) is an example of a situation where the structure of 'feeling love' becomes a part of the outsider X, who loves Y, which may be an outsider or the self. In its detector mode, the relational concept (X,empathize-structure,Y) fires when the specified X (self or outsider) empathizes in the particular way with the specified Y (self or outsider). Similarly, as a projector, this relational concept simulates such empathy.

The system can assemble a virtual outsider that serves as an **evaluator-of-the-self**. That virtual outsider analyzes the activities of the self by utilizing a specifically assembled evaluation system. Through a virtual outsider, whose detailed structure is typical to each individual, the self can experience basic feelings such as **pride, shame**, etc. These feelings result when the self is observing itself through the eyes of an outsider. The model can simulate by such a circuitry of a self-evaluator what psychologists call "super-ego".

The self's domain

With time, the basic relational concept of the **self's-domain** evolves. (,in-the-self's-domain,A), where 'A' stands for an item located in the self's domain. Outsiders that are found in certain proximity to the system, as determined by the sensory modules, satisfy the relational concept of being in the domain of the self. Even animals seem to employ the concept of 'self's-domain'. An animal may change its attitude of indifference towards objects, once they enter its self's-domain. Items that are not found in the self's domain are **out-of-self's-domain**. The 'self's-domain' and the 'out-of-domain' are mutually exclusive concepts.

5. MODELING COGNITIVE PROCESSES- AN OUTLINE

The brain performs a variety of high level mental tasks, which are made of fundamental processes. Some of the fundamental processes rely on special hardware architectures, but they are all based on the elements that were described above. This chapter deals with a variety of cognitive processes and outlines their relationships to the connectionist model presented here. Later chapters will focus on the details of some of the more common processes.

The central thinking unit (CTU)

Thinking is one of the processes in which a representation of an information entity induces the activation of other information entities, subject to some specifications and restrictions. The original information entity is the **given**, the general specifications constitute the definition of the **problem**, and the induced entity constitutes the **solution**. The given and the solution are represented by activated nodes. The modulation-factors are the main tool for encoding the specifications and restrictions of the problem.

Simple thinking processes are merely information retrieval operations. The outcome of the retrieval may be an old concept or a novel information entity, which is not yet represented in the system. Advanced thinking processes go beyond retrieval. These processes involve the projectors of the arenas. The projectors simulate situations based on the specification of the problem. Some of these situations cannot be considered 'stored information', because they have been generated for the first time during the simulation. These novel situations may be intermediate or final products of the thinking assignment.

The simplest thinking processes retrieve the required information by utilizing existing settings of modulation-factors. A reflex is one example of what might be considered a simple thinking process. Advanced thinking processes may employ iterations in which modulation-factors are adjusted and new outcomes are assessed until a satisfactory solution is found. Advanced thinking processes may recruit nodes to represent items that are defined during the search.

Many similar thinking processes are routinely executed concurrently within the various modules of the system e.g., concurrent classification of input patterns by similar detectors of a module. However, the word thinking refers usually to a unique mental process–a solo process that can use information from all the modules of the system. It will be assumed here that this kind of thinking is carried out by a specialized part of the system, which will be called the central thinking unit (CTU). The CTU relies on a communication and control network that provides the necessary connections between involved data nodes from all modules.

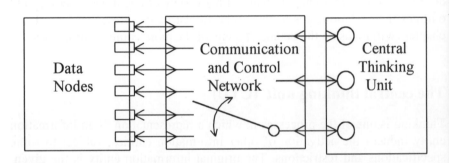

Figure 5.1: The relationships between data nodes, the communication and control network, and the central thinking unit (CTU). Nodes from the CTU (circles) can exchange signals with the modulators and the flags (rectangles) of the data nodes. The communication and control network establishes temporary connections between nodes of the CTU and the appropriate modulators and flags.

The CTU can **latch** to the nodes that represent the given. The latching ensures that the firing of these nodes is maintained as long as the system is thinking about the problem. The latching also identifies these nodes as the representation of the given. The given may include simulated events in arenas, which are generated by the projectors and analyzed by the detectors. Nodes of the CTU also activate the representations of the required relationships between the solution and the given. Those CTU nodes control the appropriate settings of the modulation-factors of the given nodes, thus representing the problem. These modulation-factors are maintained by the CTU throughout the thinking process. Based on messages from flags, the CTU finds out which active bundles of the given nodes have not invoked any responding firing nodes. These are the unmet requirements of the problem. The CTU can latch to the unmet requirements, and explicate their associations. It then can reassess the situation. If a solution is still not found, the CTU can adjust modulation factors until a solution is found, or until it declares that a solution could not be found. In the rest of the chapter, these general operations are illustrated in some important cognitive processes.

The retrieval process

A firing node can relay information through its output bundles (figure 2.3). The values of the modulation-factors of the four bundles will determine which bundles will be active, and by how much they will modulate the outgoing signals. For example, a firing node whose modulation-factor in the part-to-item bundle is 1.5, and whose other modulation-factors are zero, will send out signals of magnitude 1.5 to all its outgoing part-item synapses. No signal will propagate through any other synapse. Different combinations of modulation-factors will direct output streams from the node differently. The settings of the modulation-factors depend on the role of the node in the current task of processing information.

Information to be retrieved is often specified by the type of associations that it should have with a set of **given** entities, which are represented by nodes. If the pre-existing settings of the modulation factors of these given nodes are inconsistent with the retrieval specifications, these modulation-factors need to be modified in order to represent the retrieval request. For example, consider the instruction: invoke an exemplar of the class 'brown'. If the current settings of all the nodes have modulation-factors of one in part-to-item bundles and of zero in all other bundles, the modulation factors have to be adjusted. The modulation-factors that would represent the request are one in the class-to-exemplars bundles and zero in all other bundles. In the model, the modulation factors are controlled by signals from other specialized nodes. The latter issue instructions that adjust the appropriate factors of modulation units. Modulation instructions are elements of more general retrieval instructions.

An instruction to adjust a modulation factor of a single node or a group of nodes can originate from within the module or from other modules or units of the system. The CTU and local thinking units have specialized nodes that issue such instructions. Although they can reach nodes in all other modules, they do not need to have permanent direct connections with them. It is like a phone that can reach other phones all over the world without having permanent connections with any of them. The modulation instructions travel in a specialized **communication and control network** (figure 5.1). This network provides connections between nodes of the CTU or any localized thinking unit and the data nodes. It has relays that are switched to accommodate the nodes that need to be connected.

A thinking unit also contains nodes that receive signals from the flags of the nodes that it controls. These signals encode information about the information that is being processed by their nodes, including the firing status of the pre-synaptic and the post-synaptic nodes. This information about information, which is essential for controlling the retrieval process, reaches the thinking unit through the communication and control network.

There are several possible outcomes to a retrieval instruction including:

- The outcome of the retrieval is a node that satisfies all the required relationships with the givens. In such cases, the retrieval has been successfully completed.
- A group of nodes has been retrieved, and each member of the group satisfies, on its own, all the specifications. In such cases the retrieval instruction, which is ambiguous, is satisfied.
- Nodes have been retrieved, but none of them satisfies all the requirements. In such cases, further action may be needed. Nodes that possess the required associations, but have not been invoked because they are not contiguously associated with the givens, have to be activated by explication. This may end up in retrieving a valid solution.
- If still, none of the invoked nodes satisfies, on its own, all the requirements, but the invoked nodes as a group satisfy all the requirements, the invoked nodes constitute parts of a virtual item-node, which is a solution.
- If none of the above has occurred, a satisfactory solution could not be found.

The system has to be able to assess which of these possible situations has actually occurred, so that it can proceed in processing the information. As a first step, the system should be able to identify every unmet requirement. Unmet requirements can be identified based upon the signals provided by the flags. Then, the system should be able to regulate the modulation of its bundles and to explicate its associations, until the requirement is satisfied. If, after all that, a satisfactory node cannot be invoked, the system should be able to highlight the unmet requirement. Assessing which of the possible outcomes has actually occurred requires further analysis. A system that is unable to assess all these details can still function, but not at top performance.

Modulation adjustment

The firing of all the nodes that represent the parts of an item will cause the firing of that item node. Very often, a node that represents an item will be activated even when only some of its parts are activated. It is only required that the total activation, as relayed by the synapses of the active parts, is greater than the firing threshold of the item-node. If too few part-nodes fire, their total activation will not suffice to activate the item-node. A simple paradigm can retrieve the item-node in such circumstances, thus identifying the item to which the nodes belong. It is achieved by feedback loops that gradually increase the modulation-factors of the firing part-nodes, until an item-node fires. This process is illustrated in figure 5.2.

When the originally active group of nodes is not strong enough to activate an item-node, the thinking unit may step in. Through the modulation control units, it will keep increasing the modulation factors of the bundles, while the part-nodes are still firing. Eventually, an item-node will fire. The flags will notify the thinking unit about this event, and the search will end. In order to adjust the modulation factors in an iterative way while a solution is sought, the part-nodes have to fire continuously. If they are not activated by an external cause, the thinking unit latches to them, and keeps them firing until a solution is found. Once the flags have notified the thinking unit that there was a response from item-nodes, the unit has to check the nature of that response. If it came from one node, is this node an item node of both 'part 2' and 'part 3'? If not, that is not the solution. If 'item B' is an item node of both part nodes, is it the only item node to be retrieved? If not, does any other retrieved node contain 'part2' and 'part 3' as its parts? If yes, the solution is not unique. And so on, according to the discussion above.

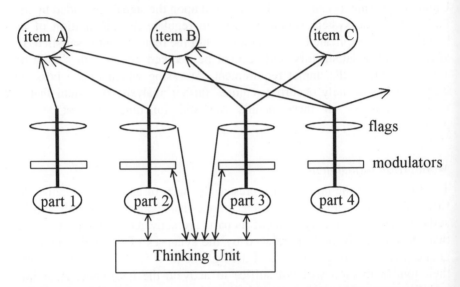

Figure 5.2: The role of modulation control in retrieval. Item-node 'item B' has three part-nodes: part 2, part 3, and part 4. The retrieval request is to 'retrieve and item whose parts are part 2 and part 3'. The thinking unit latches to 'part 2' and 'part 3', and to the modulators and flags of their part-to-item bundles. It sets the modulation factors to small values, and disables all other bundles. Then, it activates part 2' and 'part 3', while gradually increasing their modulation factors. Eventually, 'item B' will fire. That will be detected by the flags of 'part 2' and 'part 3', and reported to the thinking unit, which will terminate the search.

The iterative method described above dealt with parts that invoke their item. The same principles apply to any combination of basic retrievals (parts retrieve item, items retrieve part, exemplars retrieve class, and classes retrieve exemplar). There might be cases in which too many entities are retrieved. In such cases, the modulation factors will be decreased until only one activated entity is left.

Scanning

In scanning, a thinking unit considers a sequence of several entities, one at a time. An entity that has been considered once should not be considered again. The scanning ends when a certain condition is met, or when all possible entities have been considered. The entities to be scanned usually have a common characteristic. For example, they may all be exemplars of one class or they may be parts of one item.

The synapses from a class-node to its exemplars can have any positive weight. These synaptic weights may encode the typicality of the exemplars so that e.g., the greater the weight the more typical is the exemplar. Exemplars may then be activated one at a time, thus making them accessible for observation by the thinking unit. This can be accomplished by starting with class-to-exemplars modulation factor of zero, and increasing it gradually, while the class node is continuously firing. Exemplar nodes will be activated by descending order of their typicality. In order to have just one exemplar firing at any given time, an active exemplar node should be extinguished when a new one starts its firing. The extinguishing can be affected by linking and activating a temporary inhibitory synapse from the thinking unit to the old firing exemplar. This is one possible underlying mechanism of scanning.

Complex retrieval instructions

A complex retrieval instruction consists of the basic invoking instructions which are coupled by the logical operators AND, OR, and NOT. In general, there are many ways to actually execute a complex retrieval instruction, some of which will be discussed in a later chapter. The level of explication before executing a basic invoking operation is a variable, which must be selected by the thinking unit. Deeper explications will be needed if satisfactory solutions are not found with the initial explication levels. However, if the initial explication levels are too deep, the system may have to sift through too many possible solutions.

Manipulating the modulation factors is an important mechanism used in the execution of simple and complex retrieval requests. Circuitries that can execute a variety of complex retrieval requests will be shown in a later chapter.

Setting the ambiance

A thinking process has a group of nodes that represent the given. The problem is defined with respect to that group. In addition to the explicit given, there might be a group of nodes that represent the ambiance, or the background, in which the problem is set. The background is represented by activated nodes in the arenas. These nodes send signals to other nodes, and activate some of them to sub-threshold levels, so that the latter do not fire. As the thinking process progresses, some of these sub-threshold nodes may get additional stimulation from nodes that actually participate in the search process. Consequently, they may fire before nodes that had not received sub-threshold activation. Thus, the problem is solved within the context of its ambiance. The same problem in a different ambiance may result in a different solution.

Completion (auto association) and explication

Completion is a thinking process in which a part of an item is given, and the rest of it has to be retrieved. For example, when asked 'two plus three equals?', the given is part of the item 'two plus three equals five', and the rest of the item (five) has to be retrieved. Completion may be executed in two steps. First, the item node is retrieved ('two plus three equals five') based on some of its parts. Then, all the parts of the retrieved item are activated, including the answer-node 'five'. The first step can be accomplished by modulating the part-to-item bundles of the given nodes, until an item is retrieved. The second step is executed by modulating the item-to-parts bundle of the retrieved item. Completion does not generate new information–it just retrieves already stored one.

Completion, which is a very common element of thinking process, is sometimes executed directly, without the intermediary step of explicitly retrieving the item-node. For example, when singing a song, the next tone can be retrieved based on a few preceding tones. The preceding tones may retrieve the next tone without first retrieving the name of the song.

The difference between those two completion mechanisms is only superficial. Both of them rely on connections between parts, which encode their belonging to one item. The first completion mechanism relies on the existence of an item-node, while the second does not rely on it. However, a virtual item node may be added to the network in the second case, and participate in the completion as in the first case.

The outcome of completion is similar to that of explication, but their underlying circumstances are different. In explication, parts of an item, which are not directly connected to its item-node, become activated and may become temporarily connected to it. The item-node may inherit these parts from its class nodes or from its part nodes. Similarly, exemplar-class relationships may be explicated. Figure 5.3 illustrates some completion and explication processes:

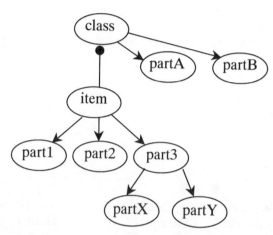

Figure 5.3: Examples of completion and explication processes. If part1 and part2 are active, they activate 'item' (by modulation), which activates part3. This is completion. When part3 activates partX and partY, and they become recognized as parts of 'item', this is explication. When 'item' activates 'class', which activates partA and partB, this is also explication, because 'item' inherits them as its parts. Temporary connections that may be established between 'item' and partX, partY, partA, and partB are not shown.

Formulas and substitution

Switching

Switching is a basic mental process that operates on elements of information structures. In switching, a member of an information structure, which is also an exemplar of a class, is replaced by another exemplar of the same class.

The new member retains all the replaced member's relationships with the rest of the information structure. The rest of the information structure is unaffected by that basic switching operation. A number of switching operations may be applied to the same information structure and affect different elements of it. Switching may include scanning operations, in which exemplars of the same class are switched one after the other until some desired outcome is obtained.

Figure 5.4 illustrates the switching operation. The dashed lines indicate the information structure. For convenience, one of its elements is shown outside the structure. Left side: the original database; right side: after a switching operation.

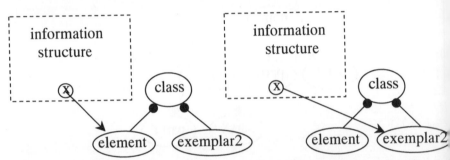

Figure 5.4: Switching operation. Node x is a part of an information structure. Its part node 'element' is switched with the node 'exemplar2'.

Formulas

In mathematics, a formula consists of a fixed set of operations and o variables. The formula operates on constants that are substituted for it variables. Similarly, in the model, a fixed circuitry that can operate or various nodes that become connected to it will be called a **formula**. The nodes which are connected to the formula are said to be the **constants**. A formula has two kinds of nodes: permanent nodes, and variable-nodes or slots. In substitution, constant nodes are connected to the slots. If a constant is connected to the slot by a bi-directional tie of unit weights, the variable and the slot becomes functionally identical–whatever activates the constant node will activate the variable node, and vice-versa. If the constant i connected to the slot as an exemplar, the two are not functionally identica but the constant still inherits the parts of the slot.

The circuitry of the formula may serve as a template, or a prototype, so that it can be duplicated and deployed in the system wherever needed. That makes it possible for the system to use the same formula concurrently in different applications. Duplicates become exemplars of a class node that represents the formula. Figure 5.5 illustrates this situation.

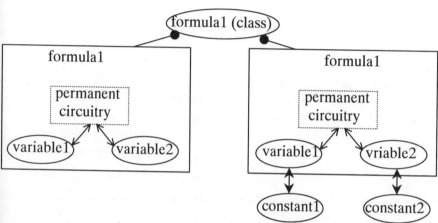

Figure 5.5: A template of a formula (left), and one of its instances (right).

Formulas usually have sub-circuitries, which will be called **bouncers**. A bouncer is a detector that checks if a substituted constant satisfies certain conditions, such as belonging to a pre-determined class. If an attempt is made to substitute an unqualified constant, the bouncer fires a node to indicate the attempt, and points to the culprit.

Abstraction and specification

Abstraction is a basic mental process. In abstraction, an information structure invokes another structure to which it is associated through the exemplar-class relationship. In simple abstractions, a single exemplar-node invokes its class-node. In more complex abstractions, exemplar-nodes in a structure invoke their class nodes in another structure. The relationships between the nodes in the exemplars' structure are mapped onto the classes' structure. For example, the information structure 'an airplane flies from New-York to Tel-Aviv' is abstracted to the structure 'object moves from point A to point B', as shown in figure 5.6. Dashed lines indicate the abstracted structure.

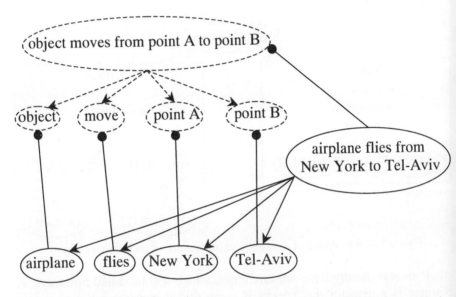

Figure 5.6: An information structure (solid lines) and its abstracted structure (dashed lines). Individual nodes of the original information structure are abstracted into nodes that are parts of the abstracted structure.

Specification is the inverse process of abstraction. In figure 5.6, this will change the abstract statement 'object moves from point A to point B' into the specific statement 'an air plane flies from New-York to Tel-Aviv'. In general, in specification, an information structure serves as a template so that its nodes guide other nodes to form a similar structure. Those other nodes are exemplars of the guiding nodes.

The roles of languages

Communicative and internal languages

Communicative languages (e.g. spoken and sign languages) enable us to describe situations that involve the environment and ourselves. Situations are described by combinations of basic concepts, which are the words of the language. Simple situations are described by a phrase or by a sentence. Complex ones are described by sequences of sentences. Sentences that describe a situation invoke its corresponding representation in our brain. Connections that exist between the invoked representation and other recorded information enable us to explore implied consequences of the situation.

The primary purpose of communicative languages has been to facilitate communication between individuals. However, we routinely rely on the analytical and abstraction powers of communicative languages to better grasp our circumstances. We quite often use communicative language in thinking processes, which are entirely internal and do not involve any communication with others.

In addition to communicative languages, the brain describes and analyzes situation by using internal representations that are not expressed by communicative symbols. Animals, including humans, use those concepts of their internal language to analyze situations as represented in their brains. Some of the internal concepts that are used are either innate or have been built from innate concepts according to innate mechanisms. In animals, frequency of co-occurrence of concepts and direct associations with rewards or adverse feelings determine how complex concepts are constructed from simple ones.

Human communicative languages adopt concepts of the internal language, which become the basic concepts of the communicative language. The adoption of concepts is determined mostly by general needs. For example, horseman tribes have many more words to describe a galloping horse than other societies. Internal concepts that are not needed for communication do not become concepts of the communicative language. Humans construct complex conceptual structures from the adopted internal concepts. These conceptual structures do not have to reflect physical realities, and they do not rely on the frequency of co-occurrence of concepts or on direct association with rewards or adverse feelings.

Communicative languages enable us to exchange information structures with other humans. Thus, information structures that were developed by one individual become part of the database of another. These structures can be decomposed into the concepts of the internal language. They can be handled and manipulated by the internal system.

Statements in a communicative language invoke internal representations in the brain. Various types of relationships may exist between a communicated statement and its corresponding internal representation. An ambiguous communicated word invokes several different internal concepts (e.g. the word 'glass'). However, a sentence that contains ambiguous words may invoke a unique representation. The brain uses the context of ambiguous words and recorded information to invoke one consistent representation. On the other hand, different communicated sentences may invoke the same internal representations. For example, the communicated statements 'John sold the car to Jane' and 'Jane bought the car from John' have the same internal representation.

An internal representation that is invoked by a communicative statement may or may not correspond to a unique real-life experience. For example, the invoked internal representation 'a bird flies in the sky' may not represent any particular event. It may invoke a generalization of many real events. Internal representations can be invoked also by real-life events. In such cases, they contain internal structures that describe the unique event. For example, when we see a dove flying, the nodes that represent this event correspond to a unique event. In addition, other co-activated nodes, such as those that represent the generalization 'a bird is flying', represent an information entity, which is related to real-life events, but not in a unique way.

Statements of the internal language describe spatio-temporal patterns of active nodes. A situation is divided into a sequence of 'snap shots' or 'frames'. The internal language groups active nodes within each frame. It also details how the active nodes participate in various relational concepts. This includes relational concepts within frames and across different temporal frames. These statements may be translated into statements of communicative languages, if the communicative languages have all the necessary words.

Categories of statements

Statements that deal with the **existence** or the **presence** of patterns of concepts constitute a major category of internal-language statements. External stimuli that activate nodes that represent concepts express the idea that these concepts are present in the scene. Detectors parse the patterns of activated nodes. Concepts that are present are delineated, and relationships between them are uncovered. Class nodes are activated by their existing exemplars. The elementary statements expressed by internal sentences are of the type: 'A is present', or 'relationship R exists between the present concepts B and C'. A, B, C and R can be innate concepts, but usually they are acquired concepts, that carry with them an entire information structure of atomic and relational concepts. Some of the nodes of these structures fire, some are primed i.e. are activated below their firing threshold, while others remain unaffected. Named concepts, i.e. concepts that are associated with words of a communicative language, are ready to be picked up by the communication module and translated into communicative sentences. The communication module constructs sentences that correspond to picked-up internal nodes.

An internal representation may be described by a variety of communicative statements. For example, 'I see rain', 'It rains', 'drops of water are falling down' etc. are the communicative outcomes of the same internal situation.

Presence statements that are invoked by external stimuli deal with the present time. Presence statements that deal with the past or with the future involve memory records of concepts. Special concepts that indicate the time convey the idea of past or future.

A second major category of statements in the internal language involves **thinking operations**. The brain directs actions of the body in response to external stimuli. It first searches a possible response that should achieve a certain goal. Potential responses are evaluated. If a possible response appears to satisfy the constraints, it is accepted and its execution is enabled. Otherwise, another response is sought, or the search is stopped altogether. Some of these processes are named, and can be expressed in communicative form. Others involve unnamed or unconscious concepts. For example, before crossing a street we watch for incoming traffic. When a car is moving in our direction, the internal system evaluates the situation. Based on the distance to the car, its perceived velocity, the distance that we have to cross, the urgency of the crossing etc., the system issues a final conclusion: 'cross' or 'do not cross'. The final statement 'cross' may have an additional qualifying concept: 'at normal pace' or 'fast'. We are not aware of the details of the thinking processes that have lead to the conclusion. They may have utilized projection operators in the visual arena. A blob that represents the approaching car might have been projected in the self's coordinate system of the visual arena. Another blob, simulating the approaching other side of the street due to our motion towards it might have also been projected. Detectors were evaluating the simulated scene. If the blob of the car came too close to the self's-range before the simulated completion of the crossing, a danger detector would be tripped, leading to the conclusion 'do not cross'. If crossing the street was urgent, the outcome 'do not cross' would not be acceptable. A new search would start, this time simulating us running across the street. The outcome of this process could be 'cross fast' or 'do not cross, cannot find a satisfactory solution'.

We cannot describe in a communicative language all the details of such underlying thinking processes. The most we could say is 'we felt that it was safe to cross' or 'we felt that it was unsafe to cross'. It might be possible, though, to train individuals so that they become aware of some of their thinking processes. Concepts that correspond to detectors that might be participating in the thinking process are defined by utilizing a communicative language. Once these detectors are named, it should be easier to notice their activation. Here are some examples of detectors that possibly participate in this thinking process. 'The car was very far and I estimated that by the time I cross the street it will still be far'. 'The car was so close that the idea of crossing scared me'. 'I was in no hurry, so why not wait'. 'The car was close but it was going slow'. 'The car was far but it was going fast'. 'The car was close and it was going fast'.

It should be noted, though, that these concepts are defined with the aid of a communicative language. We cannot be sure that the innate thinking process is based on these same concepts. Adding these concepts to the vocabulary of the internal language may replace the original unconscious thinking process with a different conscious one.

Some thinking processes utilize unconscious concepts, which are not accessible to the awareness module. Because we are unaware of the processes, we cannot name them, and they cannot be described in a reliable manner by a communicative language. They are still represented internally like any other concept, and they participate in thinking processes like any other concept. Unconscious constraints may affect the outcome of consciou thinking processes. The system may compromise a cognizable constraint in favor of a unconscious one. That would create inexplicable behaviors that are the source of confusion, frustration, and internal conflicts.

A third major category of statements are those that **create or modify information structures**. Internal languages construct their structures to reflect experiences of the self in its environment. Communicative languages can do that, and in addition they can create and modify structures in complete detachment from reality. When information is communicated to us through a communicative language or through other human communication media such as movies, cartoons, silent movies, theater, mime, etc. we translate it into internal representations. Nodes are recruited to represent the various subjects of the plot. Information structures are attached to these nodes to represent features conveyed through the communication medium. Projectors in various modules are used to simulate the activities of the objects. Detectors, which are triggered by these stimulated nodes, induce our reactions to the communicated information. All these processes, which are initiated by input in the form of a communicative language, can cause changes in records that store information.

Conflicts

Mutual exclusiveness and conflicts

The brain routinely encounters new problems that it has to solve based on its previous experiences. Consequently, new information entities, which are related to old ones, have to be created and processed. Nodes that represent new entities are related to old ones by the standard connections, which relate parts with items and classes with exemplars. Overall, new entities are created and incorporated in the modules by utilizing the basic recruiting and association operations.

While in animals new information entities represent new experiences that the animal has had in its natural environment, in humans the source of new information is often other humans. We receive from other humans processed information, which may be unrelated to or inconsistent with any real natural event. In many cases, such information is incorporated into our database, and is used by us to solve new problems that we encounter. This is one of the reasons that the brain needs means to identify and to handle incoming information or activity plans that contradict recorded information.

One of the fundamental feelings of the brain is the feeling of **conflict**. Certain things cannot happen together, and any attempt to represent them as if they do, invokes the sensation of conflict. For example, based on the brain's experiences, an object can move to the right, to the left, upwards, or downwards. An object can move to the right and upwards at the same time, but it cannot move to the right and to the left at the same time. If we are told that 'a car was moving to the right and to the left at the same time', we would feel that there is a conflict in that information piece.

New information, received from other humans or generated by the brain based on old information, may be in conflict with recorded information. The system has the capability to detect such conflicts. Once detected, the system may decide to cancel the newly conflicting information, to ignore it, or to re-evaluate the entire situation. Detection of conflicts is a fundamental property of the system. The following is one way in which it can be realized.

In order to be able to represent the occurrence of conflicts, the concept of **mutual exclusiveness** has to be embedded into the system. Various groups of entities can posses the property of being mutually exclusive: In addition to regular classes, there are also classes that are mutually exclusive. Mutually exclusive classes have all the properties of regular classes. On top of that, a group of mutually exclusive classes cannot have a common exemplar. For example, 'wet skin pixel' and 'dry skin pixel' are two mutually exclusive classes. A skin pixel cannot be an exemplar of both at the same time. Similarly, mutually exclusive items cannot have a common part; mutually exclusive parts cannot belong to one item; and mutually exclusive exemplars cannot belong to the same class.

A simple conflict occurs when one information entity is assigned to several mutually exclusive entities. For example, hot stars and cold stars are two mutually exclusive classes. The statements 'A white dwarf is a cold star' and 'A white dwarf is a hot star' are conflicting, because the exemplar 'white dwarf' cannot belong to both classes. The statements 'A white dwarf is a hot star' and 'A red giant is a cold star' are not conflicting. Whether they are factually correct or not is a different question. (They are correct).

Detection of conflict

The system has specialized detectors for detecting conflicts. These detectors monitor groups of mutually exclusive entities, and they fire whenever a conflict that involves their entities occurs. Figure 5.7 illustrates two typical situations that are handled by a conflict detector. It illustrates the peculiar property of conflict detectors. Their firing depends not only on nodes by which they are directly activated, such as class1 and class2 (**parent nodes**). The firing of conflict detectors depends also on the activation patterns that

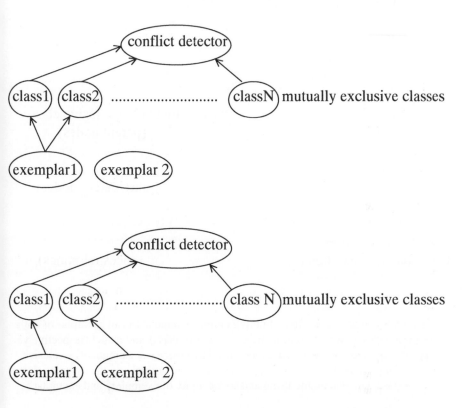

Figure 5.7: Conflict detectors. Arrows indicate possible directions of information flow. The upper figure shows a situation in which the conflict detector fires due to the activation of exemplar1, which attempts to be an exemplar of two mutually exclusive classes. In the lower figure, the conflict detector should not fire, even if exemplar1 and exemplar2 are firing, because no conflict is happening. In both cases, nodes class1 and class2, which are directly connected to the conflict detector, are firing. In line with the previous example, class1 may stand for hot stars, class2 for cold stars, exemplar1 for white dwarfs, and exemplar2 for red giants.

have caused the parent nodes to fire, such as exemplar1 and exemplar2 (the **grandparent nodes**). Since class nodes have synapses only to direct exemplars, mutually exclusive classes may have a conflicting common exemplar that is not directly connected to them. In such cases, the conflict detector has to consider firing patterns beyond the grandparent nodes, (the **ancestral nodes**), as illustrated in figure 5.8.

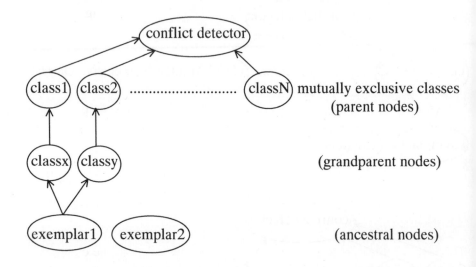

Figure 5.8; Ancestral conflicts: In this example, exemplar1 is an exemplar of both classx and classy, which, in turn, are exemplars of class1 and class2 (respectively). The nodes class1 and class2 are recognized by the system as mutually exclusive classes. The decision of the conflict detector is based not only on the firing of class1 and class2, but also on the firing and connectivity of exemplar1 and exemplar2.

A possible mechanism of relaying 'ancestral' information through several 'generations' of nodes could be by utilizing temporal encoding. If the firing of a parent node has a temporal fingerprint, and if this temporal fingerprint is found also in its children's firing, ancestral information has been relayed. Eventually, these signals will reach the mutually exclusive nodes that directly affect the conflict detector. Because of that temporal correlation, the overall effect on the conflict detector will be greater than that of un-correlated activities that would result from two different initiators (exemplar1 and exemplar2). This difference would enable the conflict detector to distinguish between conflicting and non-conflicting statements.

Topologically, when the node of a conflict detector becomes a part of a closed loop of nodes, there is a conflict in the database. For example, in figure 5.8, the closed loop, which contains a conflict, consists of the nodes: conflict detector, class1, classx, exemplar1, classy, class2, and back to conflict detector. A closed loop does not exist in the lower figure, which does not contain a conflict. This fact can be exploited for detecting conflicts that consist of any combination of the basic relationships item-part and class-exemplar.

In the model, the simulation program is responsible for detecting conflicts. It may base its decisions on labeled signals or on closed loop topologies.

Whether the system uses temporal encoding or closed loops for identifying conflicts, all the involved nodes have to be real. Virtual nodes have to be represented by real nodes, so that conflicts associated with them could be detected.

Thinking patterns

Thinking is quite often synonymous with solving problems. In the context of the model, solving a problem is a type of retrieval process that has three components: the given, the goal, and the solution. The given of the problem is a provided information structure. The goal is expressed as a general retrieval instruction, which specifies how another information structure, the solution, has to be related to the given. The solution of a thinking process may be an existing information structure, or a new structure that the system assembles according to the specifications of the goal. An implied part of thinking is that the solution should not conflict constraints that the system already has, even if those constraints are not formulated explicitly as part of the problem. However, a problem may specifically contain instructions to override constraints that the system imposes by default.

The given is expressed as a set of active nodes. The system latches them so that they are not modified in the process. The active given nodes may partially activate other nodes, which constitute the ambiance of the problem. When a solution is searched, the ambiance nodes have a head start over other nodes, which are not partially activated. In addition to the ambiance, any solution will have to comply with the 'standing rules' of the system. An acceptable solution should not create conflicts, as encoded by various circuitries of the system. The system uses the basic invoking operations, their negations, and information structures that consist of the system's concepts to define the relationships between the given and the solution. The system utilizes the basic detectors and constructors to arrive at a solution, and to evaluate it. The system may arrive at a solution in steps. It first finds structures that satisfy some of the goals of the problem. It may latch to them, and continue its search for additional structures that will satisfy the rest of the requirements. The system has means to decide which requirements are satisfied, left unsatisfied, or are conflicted by a retrieved or a newly constructed structure. In the process of solving a problem, several potential solutions may be considered by the system before a viable one is found. The system may generate these possible solutions by various strategies. Some of these strategies, such as generalized reflexes, analogical reasoning, and abstraction-specification, and the ways that they are constructed from the system's basic elements, are described next.

Generalized reflexes

In a simple reflex, a certain feature combination of an incoming stimulus causes the activation of associated nodes, usually in the motor or the feeling modules. A generalized reflex, which is a common thinking mechanism, can be viewed as a generalization of a simple reflex. In a generalized reflex, certain relationships between activated nodes and nodes of the database elicit modification of connections between other nodes. A generalized reflex involves three related information structures: the **input structure (variable) A**, a reference **database structure (fixed) B**, and an **affected structure C**. When a generalized reflex is implemented, an information entity **A**, which is associated in a prescribed way with the information entity **B**, causes changes in connections that involve the information entity **C**. The types of the prescribed associations between **A** and **B** and between **A** and **C** may vary from one generalized reflex to another.

For example, the situation described as 'if it tastes like a pizza and smells like a pizza, it is a pizza' is an implementation of the generalized reflex 'if **A** contains **B** as a part, then **A** is an exemplar of **C**'. The input **A** is an item node whose parts **B** are the taste and the aroma of pizza. The item-node **A** may represent a new event, which is happening for the first time. The system deduces that **A** is an exemplar of the class **C** (the class 'pizza'), based on the relationships that **A** has with the recorded concepts represented by **B**. In this case, noticing that the input **A** contains as its parts elements of the database **B**, acts as a generalized stimulus. It elicits a generalized response that affects connections between nodes **A** and **C**. The input node **A** becomes an exemplar of node **C**. Another example of a generalized reflex is 'if **B** is a part of **A** then **C** is a part of **A**'. For example, (in the mind of a safari participant) 'when night falls on the savanna, predators roam around'. The input variable **A** in this case is the entity 'the savanna'. When night (**B**) becomes a part of the savanna (**A**), roaming predators (**C**), too, become a part of it. In other generalized reflexes, **A**, **B**, and **C** may have many elements with a variety of relationships among them.

A generalized reflex combines a detector circuitry, which detects certain relationships, and a constructor circuitry, which manipulates connections between nodes.

Analogical reasoning

Terminology

Processes of analogical reasoning are based on the premise that if two things are similar in some respects, they will probably be similar in others. Analogical reasoning narrows the field where solutions are sought to a problem at hand, by directing the search to similar situations. Analogical reasoning has features that are found in other thinking processes, which rely on previous experiences to solve new situations. The differences are mainly a question of measure. In analogical reasoning, the similarities between the new situation and the old experience may not be as robust as in other thinking processes, and the inferences rely on procedures that are more elaborate. In addition, in analogical reasoning, the identity of the previous experience is stated explicitly, while in some other thinking processes it may be unknown.

Analogical reasoning is routinely used by the brain to find solutions to new problems based on pervious experiences. The new problem is called **the target**, and the relevant previous experience is called **the source.** The target and the source are represented in the model by information structures, each having the regular nodes and connections. In solving the problem, first, an analogical mapping is established between some of the nodes of the source and some of the nodes of the target. Then, **analogical inferences** are made:

Connections that involve nodes of the target are generated based upon existing connections that involve nodes of the source. It should be noted that an analogical inference is a mechanism to derive a potential solution to a problem. It does not guarantee that the derived inference would be a valid solution.

The model supports a variety of analogical reasoning processes. Its data structures are amenable to such processes, which can be formulated as combinations of the model's basic operations. These basic operations include 'find a class of', 'find an exemplar of', 'find a part of', 'switch', and other standard operations of retrieving data, which were discussed above. Due to the many details that are involved in analogical reasoning processes, an example of such a process will be given first. The example illustrates how the way that information is stored in the memory makes it accessible to the operations of analogical reasoning, which are expressed by the fundamental operations of the model.

Example

A common example of analogical reasoning is its use in inferring from properties of water flow to assumed properties of heat flow. Water in a pipe flows on its own from a high point to a low point. When water and heat are treated as analogs, one may infer that heat flows on its own from a hot point (high temperature) to a cold point (low temperature). In this case, the source is the available data structure pertaining to water flow. The goal is to expand the existing target's data structure, which represents the knowledge about heat, so that it would include the inference about heat flow. Figure 5.9 shows a scheme of a network that represents initial knowledge about water and heat (solid lines). It also shows an analogical inference that was made (dotted lines) based on these information structures.

It is interesting to note that the concepts of the source in this case are 'grounded' to sensory nodes in the visual arena. The more advanced concepts are related explicitly to fundamental concepts. On the other hand, 'heat' is not a fundamental concept of any arena. It can be 'grounded' to fundamental concepts of a number of modules, but this is not done here. The concept 'heat', as presented here, is floating.

The process of analogical reasoning is a sequence that consists of basic retrieval operations and constructors, which have been introduced above. The goal is to find some statement about heat flow. This means to find a concept that 'heat flow' is one of its parts. Such a concept does not exist in the database (Figure 5.9). Therefore, analogical reasoning is employed. The numbers 1-7 indicate the order in which nodes in the data structure were retrieved. First, a class node that contains 'heat flow' as its exemplar is

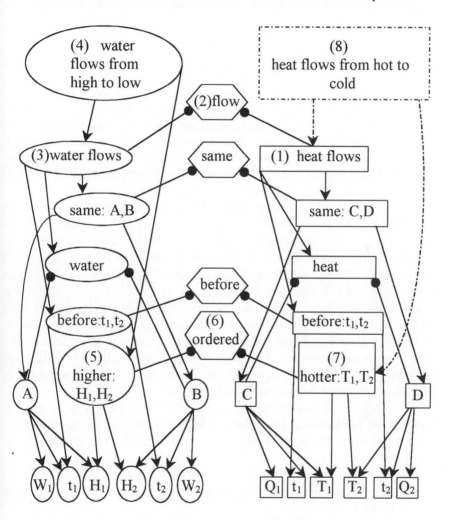

Figure 5.9: Data structures in analogical reasoning. The data structure consists of three main parts: the source (elliptical) nodes, the target (rectangular) nodes, and common nodes (hexagons). A and B are two item nodes that have been stimulated by the same water at two different times. C and D are two item nodes that were stimulated by heat at two different times. Each of these nodes has part-nodes that

represent its properties. 'W' represents water-properties, 't' represents time, 'H' represents height, 'Q' represents heat, and 'T' represents temperature. Index '1' indicates initial property, and index '2' final property. The properties of the nodes are detected by the detectors of their arena and are recorded by nodes and connections. It is recorded that: H_1 was higher than H_2; T_1 was hotter than T_2; t_1 was before t_2; 'A' and 'B' are exemplars of the class 'water', 'C' and 'D' are exemplars of class 'heat'; 'A' and 'B' are the same object; 'C' and 'D' are the same object. The parts of the concept 'water flows' indicate that the same entity 'water' was at two different points at two different times. Similarly, the parts of the concept 'heat flows' detail heat flow. The parts of the concept 'water flows from high to low' detail its elements. All the common nodes (hexagons) are class nodes, each having an exemplar in the source structure (circle) and another exemplar in the target structure (rectangle). The numbers in some boxes (1 through 8) indicate the order of the steps of the analogical reasoning process. The inferences derived by analogical reasoning (recruited nodes and connections) are denoted by broken lines.

retrieved (2). This is the concept 'flow'. Then, another exemplar of 'flow' is retrieved (3). This is the concept 'water flow'. That makes 'water flow' to become the analog of 'heat flow'. Next, an item that contains 'water flow' as its part is retrieved (4). This is the concept 'water flows from high to low'. This is the potential analog to the target. A part of 'water flows from high to low' is retrieved (5). This part is the concept 'H_1 greater than H_2', meaning initial height was greater than final height. The analog of 'H_1 greater than H_2' is retrieved, via their common class 'ordered' (6), (7). This is the concept 'T_1 is hotter than T_2'. These are analogs because they are exemplars of the same class (ordered entities). The concepts 'heat flows' and 'T_1 is hotter than T_2' recruit an item node to represent them as its part (8). This item node is the desired inference 'heat flows from hot to cold'.

This process of analogical reasoning can be expressed as a general sequence of fundamental operations, which can operate on any arbitrary target and source. The number of each step corresponds to its number in the example (figure 5.9):

(1) Let 'T'' denote any arbitrary target. (in figure 5.9 'T' was 'heat flows')
(2) Find a node 'class of T' that contains T as its exemplar. (flows in 5.9)
(3) Find a node 'analog of T', which is another exemplar of 'class of T'. (water flows in 5.9)

(4) Find a node 'analog of inference', which contains 'analog of **T**' as its part. (water flows from high to low in 5.9)

(5) Find a node 'partS', which is a part of 'analog of inference'. (H_1 higher than H_2 in 5.9)

(6) Find a node 'class of partS', which contains 'partS' as its exemplar. (ordered in 5.9)

(7) Find a node 'partT', which is another exemplar of 'class of partS'. (T_1 hotter than T_2 in 5.9)

(8) Recruit an item node whose parts will be 'partT' and '**T**'. This is the desired analogical inference. (heat flows from hot to cold in5.9)

This has been one example of an analogical reasoning process. Other sequences of the basic operations, which are assembled along the same lines, will form other analogical reasoning processes. In general, analogical reasoning would succeed to achieve its goal if a requested node is found in each of its steps. If a step cannot end up with finding a node, the process must stop, and a different sequence has to be tried.

The three basic steps in analogical reasoning as implemented by the model are: (1) Mapping between the source and the target is done by **matching exemplars of the same class** (e.g. from step 1 to step 3 in figure 5.9). One exemplar is part of the source structure, and the other is part of the target structure. (2) Expanding: Identifying potential analogical nodes, beyond the initial matching of step 1. Item or class nodes of the matched nodes are invoked (e.g. step 4). Parts of the expanded nodes are also identified (e.g. step 5). (3) Analogical mapping of the nodes identified in step 2 and inferring (e.g. steps 6-8).

Similar analogical reasoning processes can be used to derive inferences about heat from source statements about water. Here are few examples:

- The rate of water flow through a pipe increases if the height of the water source is increased. The analog is: the rate of heat flow through a heat conductor increases if the temperature of the heat source is increased.
- The rate of water flow through a pipe increases if the cross sectional area of the pipe is increased. The analog is: the rate of heat flow through a heat conductor increases if the cross sectional area of the heat conductor is increased.
- Water flows by itself from a higher point to a less high point. The analog is: Heat flows by itself from a colder point to a less cold point.

- Water is an entity that has weight. The analog is: Heat is an entity that has weight.

While these four inferences are valid analogs of factually true sources, only the first two inferences are factually true. The third and fourth inferences are factually false.

During the entire process of analogical reasoning, the target has to remain latched. The program should not 'forget' the target during the entire sequence of the retrievals, because eventually the target has to be connected with the inferred nodes.

It may happen that a concept from the target has many analogs in the source, or vice versa. There is no unique way of choosing the most appropriate analog in such cases. In general, an analog that is associated with the largest number of nodes in its structure (target or source) may be more relevant than an analog that is associated with only few concepts. Highlighting, or priming, may serve as a mechanism to mark nodes according to their degree of association with active nodes of the structure. Highlighting is a process by which active nodes send sub-threshold signals to other nodes, thus priming them. Those primed nodes have lower retrieval thresholds than unprimed nodes. Nodes that are more primed will be retrieved before less primed ones.

Abstraction- Specification

Abstraction-specification is a widely used thinking strategy. After the nodes that represent the problem are latched, they are abstracted. The abstracted entity is then expanded, usually by auto-association, and then constants are substituted into it to provide the final specific solution. The following example illustrates how abstraction-specification is employed several times in the course of solving a problem.

Consider, as an example, the situation where at dinner you want the butter, which is on the far side of the table. The given consists of the dinner table, the diners, the butter, yourself, and the rules of etiquette. The goal is to cause the butter to get to you, without violating the table etiquette. When needed, the physical objects are simulated by blobs in the various arenas. The solution would be any information structure in which the blob that represents the butter moves from the representation of the far side of the table to the representation of your domain, without violating the etiquette.

First, your mind simulates reaching the butter by yourself. Projectors in the arenas project the blob of your hand moving towards the blob of the butter. But it stops short. The butter is a little too far. Then, your mind may simulate another possible solution: reaching the butter using the long fork from the central salad bowl. The blobs of the fork and the butter meet, all right, but a detector circuitry that detects violations of etiquette-rules fires. That circuitry may be quite complex. It encodes the concept that using any table utensil not for its designated purpose is a violation.

Finally, your mind realizes that the blob of the person next to the butter may move the blob of the butter into the blob of your spatial domain. This could be initiated by you saying 'would you please pass the butter'. Finding such a solution is the result of a sequence of abstraction-specification processes, one of which is illustrated in figure 5.10. It starts by latching the

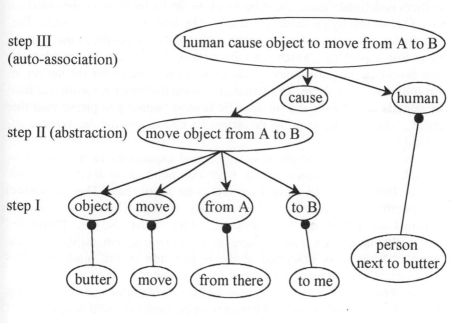

Figure 5.10: Steps in an abstraction-specification thinking process.

goal 'the blob of butter moves next to myself'. Then, the system looks for an abstracted form of the goal. The elements of the goal invoke their class nodes (step I in figure 5.10). An item, whose parts are these classes, is searched and found. This is the entity 'object moves from point A to point B' (step II in the figure). This statement, which is an abstraction of the goal, is then expanded by auto-associated. Another statement by which it is contained is invoked. The expanded statement is 'human cause object to move from one point to another' (step III in the figure). This structure is then made specific. It is treated as a formula, and all its exemplar-class ties are replace by bi-directional unit weight, resulting in the substitutions of the constants. 'Butter' is substituted for 'object'. 'The location of the butter' is substituted for 'from point A'. 'Next to me' is substituted for 'to point B', and 'the person next to the butter' is substituted for 'human'. Thus, a possible solution is found: person next to butter cause butter to move from its current place to me.

After noticing that the person does not pass the butter, a secondary problem is defined: 'cause the person next to the butter to move the butter to me'. This secondary problem is also solved by abstraction-specification. The information structure 'asking a human to do something results in that human doing that something', which is an abstraction of the secondary problem, is then invoked. The person next to the butter is substituted for the human in that information structure. The action of moving the butter is substituted into the general action slot, and the specific request 'would you please pass the butter', which is the name of the action, is substituted for the variable of general request.

There are other possible abstractions and expansions to the goal. For example, 'the wind blows objects from one point to another' instead of 'human cause object to move from one point to another'. This possibility was not invoked because of the ambiance setting. 'Human' is partially activated as a part of the ambiance, while 'wind' is not. Therefore, statements that contain 'human' have head-start over statements that contain 'wind'. The process described above is just one of the many possible processes. This processes relied on the way that data is recorded in the memory, and on the standard processes of retrieving class nodes, retrieving item nodes, and modification of connections between activated nodes.

Individualized thinking paradigms and character

Generalized reflexes, analogical reasoning, and abstraction-specifications are some of the general thinking schemes, which are used by the brain. In addition to them, individuals develop their own thinking paradigms, which consist of these general tools combined with individualized elements.

Records of thinking plans that were successful in the past are kept in the memory and are recalled when similar circumstances recur.

In general, thinking processes include steps in which the given is generalized or abstracted. There are many ways to generalize a given. One of the factors that affect the outcome of a generalization is which entities have been primed before the actual generalization. In the retrieval process, primed entities have a head-start over unprimed ones. For example, a pessimistic person primes representations of unpleasant events, while an optimist primes the pleasant ones. As a result, when provided with the same stimulus, the pessimist will call it a half empty glass, while the optimist will call it a half full. In its extreme, priming becomes downright retrieval. The outcome is automatically retrieved due to the priming, without any additional searching process.

A person's character shows itself by the ways that that person reacts in a variety of situations. These reactions depend on the thinking paradigms that the person uses, and on the primed information in the system. By selecting the appropriate thinking paradigms and the typical primed entities in the system, the model can simulate various human characters.

Conscious and unconscious thinking

The brain is capable of being aware-of some of its own processes. Therefore, in the model, awareness is detected by detectors and is represented by nodes, much like any other concept that the model employs. Awareness detectors can characterize the nature of an ongoing process and the sources of its information, e.g. external stimuli, internal processes, communicated from other individuals, and so on.

In addition to detectable processes, some processes are completely undetectable, and some are only partially detectable by awareness detectors. Thinking and learning belong to the latter group. Both detectable and undetectable circuitries participate in thinking and in learning. In some thinking processes we are completely aware how we have derived the solution to a problem. In some processes, we cannot tell, and in others, we may think that we know, but in reality, the outcome was generated by unconscious, undetectable processes.

In thinking processes, the system looks for solutions that should not be in conflict with existing constraints. If a potential solution is found and the system realizes that it is conflicting one of the constraints, the system will try to modify that potential solution. However, the system is teeming with conflicting constraints–sets of constraints that cannot be completely satisfied by any solution. Various psychological theories define the fundamental conflicts and describe the mechanisms that the system employs to address them. For example, according to Freud, the mind can be divided into three functional compartments: the id, the ego, and the super ego. The id consists of drives to satisfy innate pleasure sensations. The ego embodies realizations that planning may be needed to satisfy those needs. The super-ego contains impediments and restrictions that were imposed by parents, authority figures, and society in general on the id's drives. Sometimes, actions for immediate satisfaction have to be suppressed first and then modified in one way or another. Other psychological schools divide the mind differently, but most, if not all, would agree that the mind has to deal all the time with resolving conflicts, some of which reside in the system. The interplay between conscious and unconscious processes, and how they are represented by the model will be discussed in chapter 7.

Dreams

A number of theories have been proposed regarding the nature and purpose of dreams. Individuals often find that dreams provide solutions, or at least hints, to real life problems. Both the problems and the solutions are usually encoded by symbols borrowed from the individual's own experiences, as recorded by the brain. Individuals can sometimes decode the real life meaning of their own dreams, based on the ways that information is stored in the system. Relationships between exemplars and their class node provide a key to the encoding used by the brain. The following example of a dream and its interpretation, as told to the author by a colleague, is a case in point:

> Before I went to bed, I read in the Washington Post an article about the AIDS epidemic in South Africa: "Currently, more than sixteen percent of the population are infected with the HIV virus. ...Millions of South Africans caught in the complex and deadly web of ignorance, denial and misplaced cultural beliefs that is fueling South Africa's AIDS epidemic, which is the most aggressive on the continent.... The infection level among South Africans between the ages of 20 and 30 already is approaching 20 percent. New infections are being reported at a rate of 1,500 a day–two-thirds of them among 15- to 20-year-olds". I was

shocked. It means that in a group of five people, one might be infected with the virus. I fell asleep, and when I woke up, I remembered a dream that I had. I was going to the beach, where I met some good friends. The waves were smooth and clear, very inviting. There were some white things moving occasionally in the water. I watched closer, and realized that these were white jellyfish, of all sizes, moving elegantly and effortlessly. I asked my friend if he noticed them, and he answered. "Oh, yes, they are very stingy. I am not getting into the water, it's not worth it".

The problem of having sexual relationships during the AIDS epidemic was invoked by the newspaper's article. The dream provided a clear answer, using an individualized code. Swimming in the inviting waves symbolizes sexual pleasures. The white jellyfish symbolize the deadly HIV virus that is carried by innocent looking individuals of all sizes (ages?). The good friend is the provider of the caring advice to avoid sexual relationships, even with innocent looking people.

The semantic relationships between the entities of the problem and their symbols in the dream are simple. Key elements in the information structure of the problem were swapped with other exemplars of the same class to create the information structure of the dream. Sexual pleasures were swapped with swimming pleasures. Contact with HIV virus was swapped by the more tangible contact with white (deadly?) jellyfish. The chancy element of contracting HIV through sex was swapped with the chancy event of getting in contact with jellyfish while swimming. The friend's advice was the solution, as provided by the metaphors of the dream.

In this dream, an analogy was formed between a real life problem, the target, and the plot of the dream, which was the source. In dreams, unlike in conscious situations, the target may be un-latched. It is not saved by the system, so that an inference to reality is not provided. The inference has to be made by an external dream interpreter, which has to be able to determine what has been the target behind the dream. It is not known how the brain has constructed the source and generated the mapping between the source and the target. The proposition that the brain uses analogical reasoning procedures in dreaming provides a mechanism that is common to thinking and dreaming processes.

Learning

General Considerations

The innate system consists of the peripheral nodes and innate operator: (detectors and projectors). All the other nodes are unassigned. As the system evolves, nodes are recruited and assigned to represent various information entities. Information structures, which consist of nodes connected by the standard part-item and exemplar-class ties, are formed. The processes by which these structures are formed are the model's rendition of learning.

Learning processes, which generate internal representations of the environment and the self, employ two main procedures: First, assembling distinct entities into new wholes (items); second, recording relationships between entities. Distinct entities are assembled into new wholes through the part-item connections. Other relationships between entities are expressed through the exemplar-class connections. Based on that, the learning rules, which govern the learning processes, regulate how item nodes are defined, how parts are connected to item nodes, how class nodes are defined, and how exemplar nodes are connected to class nodes. These basic operations are used to construct new data structures, detectors, and projectors from the innate nodes and the innate operators of the system.

Due to the limited resources of the system, it must employ pragmatic strategies about what to learn and how to record it. Generally, events that repeat themselves are deemed more relevant to the existence of the system than rare events. The system, though, has to learn also some rare events, which might have high relevance to its existence. These events are usually associated with emotions, such as gratification and disappointment. Both frequent and rare events should be recorded in such a way that the system could correctly recognize them when they recur. For that purpose, the system does not have to record them in full detail. The state of every peripheral node that participates in an event need not be recorded. In fact, detectors, innate and learned, are triggered by certain feature combinations that are present in the events. Then, typical combinations of such firing detectors provide a compact way of characterizing the events. It is therefore reasonable to assume that in order to record an event, the system records which detectors it has activated. In other word, it records what familiar combinations of feature-combinations are contained in the information.

The whole purpose of recording events is to be able to distinguish between various situations. Ideally, any new event being recorded should be compared with all previously recorded events. Unique feature combinations that the event has should be identified as well as feature combinations that it shares with previously recorded events. All these feature combinations would be used to build information structures that characterize the event and define its relationships with other events. As new information structures are being constructed, the system has to be aware of possible conflicts that may result, and try to avoid them. These general principles should apply to the learning of both frequently recurring and rare events.

In neural networks theory, it is common to distinguish between two major learning paradigms–supervised and unsupervised. In supervised learning, the response of the system to a given stimulus is compared by a 'supervisor' with a desired target. Based on the match between the actual response and the target, the supervisor issues instructions to the network how to modify its ties. The supervisor may be outside of the system, or it may be another sub-unit within the system. In unsupervised learning, there is no set target against which the behavior of the system is measured and which directs its learning.

In the model, learning processes are controlled by learning units. A learning unit is responsible for performing a certain learning paradigm in a group of nodes that it controls. Activation of those nodes is sensed and analyzed by the learning unit, which then issues instructions to modify connections between the appropriate nodes. The model supports both supervised and unsupervised learning paradigms. Following are some examples that illustrate how the model handles various learning paradigms.

Classification

Parsing and classification

Parsing is an operation in which firing nodes that share common features become parts of a newly defined item-node. Such new item-nodes help the system to further analyze the scene. The system relies on innate and acquired feature detectors, which operate concurrently in the arenas, to accomplish the parsing. The most basic features that parsing can rely upon are those that are represented by nodes of pixel's-clusters. For example, in the visual arena parsing can be based on color, illumination-intensity, direction of motion, speed, etc. In the auditory module, parsing can be based on pitch, tone-quality, temporal pattern of frequency ratios, etc.

In **acute classification**, an item-node, which was defined in a parsing process, becomes an exemplar of an existing class node. This may happen when the system feels that the current event is very significant, and it should be recorded. For example, after a traumatic experience, the system records its circumstances so that it could be avoided in the future. Feature combinations of that event, as expressed by firing detectors, recruit a node to represent them through the parts-item relations. The new item-node is then connected as an exemplar to an existing class-node that represents the feeling that the event has invoked. This class-node will be activated by the firing of its new exemplar when it recurs. For example, visual patterns associated with a traumatic experience are first connected as parts to an item-node in the visual arena. This item-node, in turn, is connected as an exemplar to the class node 'danger'. Whenever these visual patterns recur, they will activate their representation in the visual arena, which will activate the 'danger' node.

In unsupervised classification feature combinations that have been appearing repeatedly in many events are joined to become parts of a new item. This item may become a pointer of a class-node. Any similar new scene will activate that class-nodes, thus signaling its resemblance to the previous events. The purpose of unsupervised-classification is to establish records of familiar situations, so that the system does not have to analyze them from the beginning every time that they recur. Items defined through unsupervised classification may establish all kinds of relationships with other items in other information structures. Detectors that are developed in unsupervised classification may act as acquired parsers. For example, when we look at a scene, we immediately parse out human shapes that it contains. Many shape-classifiers are being developed over periods of time in unsupervised processes, based on repeated experiences.

Classification rules

Classifiers are prevalent and important detectors. They classify information entities as belonging to given classes. A classifier is an information structure that has a class-node and at least one pointer-node. Any other firing item that contains that pointer will cause the activation of the classifier's class node. That will serve as an indication to the system that the item belongs to the class. Some of the classifiers are innate, but most of them are learned from experience.

The system establishes new classifiers and updates old ones through learning processes. By classifying a new item, a classifier predicts what should be the implied properties of that item. The goal of the system is that its classifiers 'correctly' classify any new event. Correctly, in this context, means that the predicted properties of the classified item should not conflict its real properties. For example, if classifiers classify an item as tasty food, eating it should not create the feelings that it is terribly bitter.

Humans develop their classifiers based on their own experiences, and based on information supplied by other humans. The main challenge to the system when it develops its classifiers based on its own experiences is to find out which feature combinations that the present item has will always point to the same class. If the system can identify these pointers, it will correctly classify any new item. At the beginning, any parsed item of a scene is a candidate to become a pointer to the current class. As new events are analyzed, some of those pointers prove to be erroneous. The system then trims them out.

There are many sets of learning rules that a system can use in order to establish and modify connections between potential pointers and class nodes. Three general principles can serve as guides in defining classification rules. First, whenever an item has been classified correctly, it makes sense to not weaken the connections between its firing pointers and its firing class-node. These connections may be left unchanged or strengthened, depending on the set of learning rules that the system employs. Second, it makes sense to weaken the connections between firing pointers and a firing class-node when the classification is erroneous. Third, there is no good reason to strengthen a connection between a firing pointer and its now quiet class-node, with which it has been associated in the past. These general principles depend only on the firing status of the involved nodes and of signals from a supervisor, which compares the prediction of the existing classifier with the real situation.

Unsupervised classifiers, which group features into items based on the frequency of their occurrence, may use some different learning rules. One of the goals of such classifications is to be able to identify groups of features that appear together. When a set of features appears in many different items, a node is recruited to represent them. This node can act as a pointer to a new class to which all these items belong. Any future item that contains this set of features will be classified as an exemplar of that class. Unsupervised and supervised classification can operate jointly on the same data, and complement each other.

The system can deploy various learning paradigms. Some of the major ones are discussed next.

Conditioning

In **classical conditioning**, an innate (unconditioned) response of an animal to a certain cue is associated with another arbitrary cue. Eventually, that arbitrary cue, by itself, would elicit the innate response. Classical conditioning is also called Pavlov's conditioning, after the famous experiments in which giving food (unconditioned stimulus) to a dog was preceded by a cue, such as a bell ring (conditioned stimulus). Eventually, the dog would salivate to the sound of the bell, even when no food was given to it (conditioned response). After that, if the bell is rung many times without giving food, it would lose its effect, and the dog would not salivate to the ring (extinction).

The model can simulate classical conditioning, assuming that there is an innate circuitry behind this process. A class-node called 'salivary gland activator' represents the neurons that activate the salivary gland. One exemplar that belongs to that class-node is a node that represents the neurons in the mouth that detect the presence of food. Due to conditioning, the node that represents the sensation of a bell-ring will become another exemplar of the class-node 'salivary gland activator'. As an exemplar, when stimulated by a ring, it will activate its class-node 'salivary gland activator', which will activate the salivary gland. The various nodes that participate in this conditioning process are shown in figure 5.11.

An innate exemplar-class connection exists from the 'food detector' to the 'salivary gland activator'. Whenever the 'food detector' fires, the 'salivary gland activator' fires too. Other innate circuitry encodes that concurrent activation of 'food detector' and 'salivary gland activator' triggers the 'was right' node. The firing of 'salivary gland activator' without the concurrent firing of 'food detector' triggers the 'unsatisfied' node (false prediction). The firing of the 'was right' node prompts the reinforcement of exemplar-class connections from the concurrently firing nodes to the 'salivary gland activator' node. That would include the 'bell sound' and the 'unrelated background' nodes. The "erroneous" connections between 'background nodes' and the 'salivary gland activator' node will be trimmed-off as a result of other experiences, in which salivation was erroneously triggered without the presence of food. Such events trigger the 'was wrong' node, which initiates the trimming.

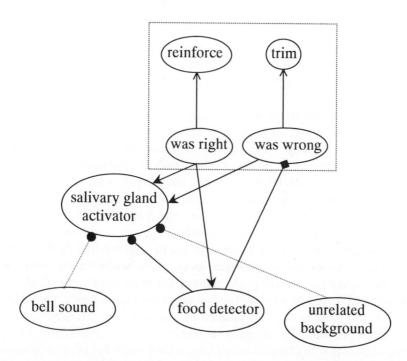

Figure 5.11: A model of a circuitry of Pavlov's experiment. The 'was right' node fires when salivation was associated with food. That happens when its parts, 'food detector' and 'salivary gland activator', fire together. The 'was wrong' fires when salivation occurred with no food present. This node is inhibited by firing of the 'food detector', and is activated when only the 'activator of salivary gland' fires. The activation of the 'was right' and 'was wrong' nodes activate the nodes that control changes of synaptic weight between active nodes. The nodes 'was right, was wrong, reinforce, and trim' constitute an internal supervisor of this learning process.

Hebbian learning is a process in which ties between two neurons that fire within the same time window are established or modified. In the conditioning example described above, the processes of establishing and modifying exemplar-class connections were Hebbian processes. They were regulated by signals from the 'reinforce' and 'trim' nodes. Signals to reinforce connections or to trim them are broadcast to certain areas, where they can regulate Hebbian learning in any pair of firing neurons. It is also possible that the system marks a selected class node ('activator of salivary gland' in the example), to which firing exemplar nodes should be attached or have their weight modified by Hebbian learning. This marking would make the learning process more focused and efficient. Concurrently firing nodes of events that are not related to the learned subject (e.g. the dog wagging its tail) should not change their connections. On the other hand, if marking is used, different learning processes could take place independently of each other at the same time.

In **operant conditioning**, an animal learns by trial and error to respond to a given cue in one of several possible ways. First, the animal is doing what it does normally. Then, an external cue and an external reward are matched with one particular act of the animal. The animal learns to associate that particular act with the external cue and with the reward. This particular act becomes the 'correct' response to the cue. The animal is rewarded only when it responds 'correctly' to the given cue. Eventually, it will execute the 'correct' in response to the cue even without getting a reward. For example, a pigeon has to peck at one of three levers in response to a flash of light. If the pigeon pecks on the correct lever, it is rewarded by some food. Eventually, the pigeon will peck on that lever in response to the flash even if no food is released. If food will not be provided anymore as a reward for the correct peck, the pigeon will unlearn its behavior. The circuitry that carries out operant conditioning is similar to that of classical conditioning. The main difference is that in classical conditioning the system learns about a stimulus and in operant conditioning it learns about a response.

The process of operant conditioning has some similarities with the human process of naming, in which names (words) are assigned to experiences. In operant conditioning, the animal has to associate the node of the correct response with the node of the cue. It has to map from one group of cue nodes (levers and light) to another group (motor activators). In naming, the mapping is between nodes that represent experiences and nodes that represent their names.

Naming

Humans can assign names to concepts that are represented by real or by virtual nodes. The name itself, which is represented by a name-node in the communication module, is a part of an information structure. The name-node has standard associations with other nodes within the communication module and in other modules. A name-node is usually connected to nodes that represent its visual and auditory symbols (figure 5.12). Activation of a name-node can originate at the auditory module, where a sound pattern that symbolizes it is picked up, or at the visual module, where an image that symbolizes it is detected. Thus, the sound and visual symbols of a name act as exemplars of their name-node. A name-node that is activated by its sound or visual symbols can activate the memory representation of the real events with which it has been associated, and it can be activated by those memories. A name-node can also be activated by the representation of its associated real event, but, generally, it cannot activate a pattern that represents the presence of a real event. All these relationships are realized by the connections between the name-node and its related nodes, as illustrated in figure 5.12. The actual information flow in the circuitry that contains a name node will depend on the setting of the modulation factors. For example, the setting of the modulation factor of the class-to-exemplar bundle of the name-node will determine if its auditory symbol (e.g. the sound of a word) will be activated when the actual event is present at the peripheral module, and is detected by the detector of the real event.

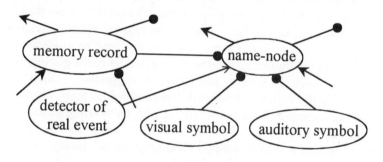

Figure 5.12: A name node and its associated nodes.

Naming is a process that associates a name-node with the nodes that represent its real-life experiences. For example, when an event gets the name 'explosion', the name-node 'explosion' is associated with the node that represents all the sensations of explosion that have been experienced in the visual and auditory arenas. If there is no item-node that represents all the parts of that event, the name-node 'explosion' assumes also the role of an item-node. The visual and auditory parts of the event belong now to a real item-node, which is also a name-node. Similarly, a name-node that represents a set of exemplars of a virtual class becomes their real class-node.

The network of the connections between related name-nodes should reflect the network that connects their associated events. Fore example, if event A is a part of event B in some peripheral module, the name-node of event A should be a part of the name-node of event B in the communication module. However, this is not a complete one-to-one-correspondence. Some events may have no name-nodes. For those who have, not all the relationships between the events are actually reflected by similar relationships between their name-nodes, and vice-versa. Many mental processes, which involve manipulation of information, utilize only name-nodes. Once a process is completed, the outcome, which is represented by certain name-nodes, can invoke its associated representation in the other modules. Similarly, mental processes can manipulate representations that are recorded only in modules other than the communication module. Once completed, the outcome can invoke its associated representation of name-nodes, if they exist. Mental processes can also utilize mixtures of name-nodes and non name-node representations of information entities.

In naming, a teacher provides the name, and the pupil's system associates it with the representation of the corresponding event. Learning names from a teacher can be a lengthy process of refining relationships between the name-node and old and new information. For example, if at the sight of a rushing ambulance, its siren blaring and its lights glaring, the word 'ambulance', which is new to the pupil, is suggested, it then becomes associated with the entire audio-visual experience. The pupil would be able to narrow the meaning of the word 'ambulance' by revising its associations, as the teacher points to a parked, off duty ambulance. In this respect, the process of learning names is similar to learning how to classify. Both depend on comparing and contrasting, and both become simpler if only relevant information is provided during the training period.

Time and order

The perceptions of time and order

Perceiving time is one of our innate abilities. The brain can characterize two events as occurring at the same time or at different times. It can distinguish between events that have occurred in the past, events that are occurring now, and events that we anticipate in the future. The brain can organize events in the order that they have occurred, or in the order that we anticipate them to occur. According to the principles of the model, it should be possible to represent temporal concepts, like any other concept, by nodes. These nodes are activated by temporal detectors, which detect when a certain temporal feature is present in an entity. The detectors may also initiate the formation of circuitry to represent detected temporal relationships. These nodes become parts of information structures, and their activation indicates that the information entity possesses the temporal feature.

Whenever humans describe events, time is treated as a feature that is attached to the main part of the event. In physics, this is referred to as the time coordinate of the event. The numerical value of the time coordinate is provided by an outside device–a clock. Two events that happen at the same time have the same value of the time coordinate. By knowing the time coordinates of events, it is possible to figure out which event happened first and which happened later, as well as other temporal relationships. An interesting question is whether this paradigm of handling time is also employed by the brain. Does the brain use some 'internal clock' that supplies time values, which are then 'time stamped' into representations of events? Are there temporal detectors that can assign temporal properties to events, based on these time stamps?

The body uses biological clocks to regulate its circadian rhythms. For example, the daily cycle of awake and sleep is regulated by such a clock. The biological correlate of time-flow in this clock is apparently the concentration levels of certain hormones, such as melatonin, in the bloodstream. Sensors of the concentrations of these hormones relay their findings to the brain, which processes them and coordinates the activities of the body. The length of the hormonal concentration cycle is synchronized from time to time by external signals, such as daylight and typical sounds. It is not known if signals from these concentration sensors are used to generate 'time stamps' for other recorded events. It is also not known if the brain has dedicated neural circuitry, which generates signals that serve as time stamps of events. Whatever the biological correlates of time sensing and 'time stamping' are, this model will treat time as a class, whose exemplars, the time values, are provided by an outside source, beyond the control of the system (for the time being...).

An important element in the perception of time is the detection of the time-order of two events. The input to a time-order detector consists of two consecutive events. The outcome consists of the formation of several ties between nodes: The first event becomes an exemplar of the class 'first events'. The second event becomes an exemplar of the class 'second events'. Both events become parts of a newly recruited node 'a pair of events', which is an exemplar of the class 'pairs of events'. The time-order detector is reset after the two events have been analyzed. If two events enter the time-order detector within a short time window, they are declared 'concurring', and become exemplars of that class. Figure 5.13 illustrates how the fact that two events, event1 and event2, that occurred consecutively is recorded in the network. Such structures are the outcome of the activity of a time-order detector.

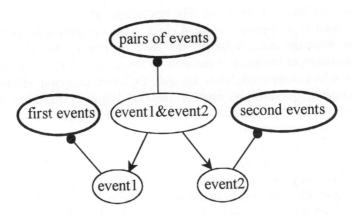

Figure 5.13: A data structure that records two consecutive events. Bold lines indicate class nodes that are used to record such events. Events are assigned to these class nodes by time-order detectors.

Time-order detectors can be stacked in an array, so that the order in which any number of events have occurred can be detected and recorded. An ordering scheme must be transitive, because time ordering is transitive by nature. If a time detector has determined that event1 happened before event2 and event 2 happened before event3, a time ordering detector should also determine that event1 happened before event3.

Combinations of time-order detectors and other detectors create the perceptions of other temporal concepts. The combination of a time-order detector and a present detector, which indicates that an event is occurring now, creates the perceptions of past, present, and future. For example, if the second event is occurring in the present, the first have occurred in the past. If the first event is occurring in the present, the second is a future event.

Time-order detectors are the most fundamental of the many order-detectors that humans use. They provide a template for defining order of other multi-valued attributes. If different values of an attribute are activated one at a time and once, and if those events are detected and ordered by time-order detectors according to the time of their occurrence, the values of the attribute become ordered too. For example, consider a muscle unit that contracts continuously starting at the relaxed state. The contraction states are represented by corresponding firing nodes. Time-order detectors can assign order to those firing nodes, according to the time that they have contracted, as in figure 5.14. Based on their time order during this particular set of events, the values of the attribute can be ordered. Such an order will become a permanent property of the node–a property that can be detected by its own order detector. Thus, the initial state of the muscle is described as the least contracted, the final state is described as most contracted, and all the contractions in between are ordered accordingly. This order, which will have its own detector, could be interpreted from now on as 'amount of contraction', although originally the events were ordered by time-order detectors. The newly established order detector relies on memory records of the original sequence of events. Figure 5.14 illustrates how time ordering is extended to ordering other attributes.

An order detector of one attribute can be used to define order of another multi-valued attribute. For example, we can raise our chin by contracting our neck muscles, an activity that is controlled by the corresponding motor neurons. The contraction will be the entity that is represented by the class 'contraction', and the different amounts of contraction will be the exemplars of that class. As we raise our chin continuously, from a low position to a high position, the increasing amounts of contraction of the neck muscles can be ordered based on the time of their occurrence. Now, assume that as we move our chin up, we look at the windows of a skyscraper. The sequence of windows that we see are parts of a set of information entities. Each entity has a visual component and a neck muscle component. The neck muscle components are ordered attribute values. Based on them, we can order the visual components of the entities, and call them low window, higher window,..., highest window.

The way that we perceive time, and especially time order, enables us to define a variety of order-detectors directly and indirectly. Time is the fundamental template by which other entities can be ordered. A common intermediary concept that is employed for ordering information entities is the concept of numbers. The sequence of integers 1, 2, 3... represents a sequence of events that are mapped in our memory as a temporal record. It is quite possible that when we reach the conclusion that 5 is greater than 3 we do it by comparing their temporal order in our basic acquired memory record of 'can you count from one to ten?' We get to 3 before we get to 5.

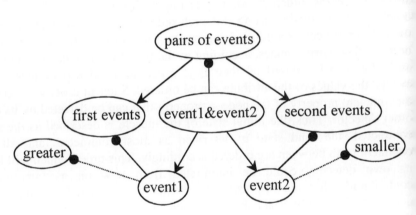

Figure 5.14: Extending order from temporal to other attributes. Greater and smaller are assigned based on a particular temporal sequence of events.

All the operations of defining and creating ordered entities rely solely on the basic operations of establishing standard ties between nodes, and recruiting new nodes to represent new information entities.

Playback, assimilating plots, and planning

An event is usually represented by a large number of firing nodes. Even if the event is instantaneous, not all its nodes will start firing at the same ime, because some nodes often cause the firing of others. Nevertheless, the system has to recognize that all the firing nodes represent one entity. If the buildup time of the firing is short compared to the time during which the entire representation is on, the system may ignore the buildup time, and perceive all the firing nodes as one event. The system may then record pertinent features of the event in its memory. To invoke the memory of this event, the system would recall these features, and keep them firing as long as the invoked memory needs to be active.

Before recording a sequence of events, the system first breaks it into instantaneous frames, and keeps a record of each one of them. The system then interweaves the frames, so that they could be played back in the right order. If frame X happened before frame Y, the system has to record that relationship by its hardware. Figure 5.14 illustrates one way of doing it. A more direct circuitry that would simplify the playback of sequences of frames relies on the concept 'is followed by' (IFB in short) being represented by its own node. The nodes X and IFB become parts of a pointer node, which point to node Y, as illustrated in figure 5.15. The activation of the node IFB when node X is active will trigger the activation of node Y. Node Y may then send an inhibitory signal to shut off node X. If frame X has to stay active concurrently with frame Y, the shut off signal will not be sent. The involvement of node IFB in the process encodes the fact that node and node Y represent a sequence of two events. This circuitry could be used as a basic building block for recording time sequences of any number of events.

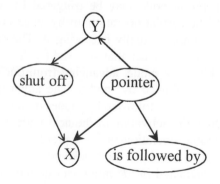

Figure 5.15: Keeping a record of a sequence of events by using the 'is followed by' concept.

The activation of IFB nodes is initiated by a controller. The timing of their activation will determine the playback speed of the entire sequence.

When we read a story or listen to someone talk, our system builds a mental picture of the high level information, which is provided to us in verbal form. The provided information is parsed into frames, which are represented in different modules, as warranted. Each frame represents information that constitutes a scene. The frames are interwoven by 'is followed by' nodes. This is an explicit way of representing the time order of the frames. In addition, frames may include projectors that simulate the time evolution of events within the scene. 'Blobs' of nodes in the arenas represent the subjects described in the story. These blobs are then hooked up, by the standard ties, to existing information structures in the memory's database. These connections create the structures that contain information related to the blobs. Projectors act on the blobs in accordance with the story, and animate them. These processes trigger our responses to the story. A similar situation occurs when we watch a movie or a show. The 'blobs', which are generated in our arenas, are associated with the characters and the objects of the plot. The thoughts and the feelings that are invoked in our mind are due to activated nodes in the information structures, which participate in the process. The recorded plots could be played back at a desired speed by appropriately timing the activation of the IFB nodes.

A plan is a sequence of operations, each of which is represented by a node. The firing of certain operation nodes initiates the actual activity of subordinate motor units. The operation nodes of a plan fire in a given order. The firing of the next operation node may be triggered by a signal that indicates the completion of the current operation, or by an external cue. The mind can playback a plan without actually executing it. The circuitry of a plan consists of core nodes, and of nodes that are used by the mind only for playing the plan back. In playback mode, advancing from one operation to the next is facilitated by 'is followed by' nodes. The advancing speed is determined by the controller. The 'is followed by' nodes do not participate in the execution mode, in which the activation of the next node is triggered by the termination of the ongoing operation or by a pre-determined cue. For example, consider the plan of going down the block and crossing the street at the corner. The plan, as constructed in the mind, can be represented by the circuitry of figure 5.16.

An operation node of a plan may represent another sub-plan. In the previous example, 'sensation of a corner' may represent a sub-plan, in which the traffic lights are detected, observed and evaluated, then the actual traffic in the street is considered, and finally, the signal 'ok to cross' is issued. The mind can playback a plan according to a desired level of details. Once the node 'sensation of a corner' is played back, the system may continue by playing back the 'cross the street' node, or by playing back of the sub-plan of analyzing the traffic at the corner. To have this flexibility, the system may use several strings of 'is followed by' nodes. Each level of detail has its own playback string.

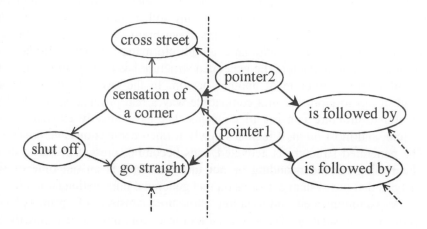

Figure 5.16: Nodes involved in an action-plan to cross a street, and in playing it back. The part of the circuitry to the left of the dashed line represents actions and sensations that are involved in the process. The part of the circuitry to the right of the dashed line is needed only for playing back the plan. The nodes 'is followed by' are activated in a sequence by the external controller (dashed arrows), which determines the pace of the playback. The nodes pointer1 and pointer2 are intermediary nodes that facilitate the playback of the plan. Only core nodes participate in the actual execution of the plan. These nodes are shown to the left of the dashed line.

Understanding

Understanding as a feeling

We can tell when we understand information that was communicated to us by other humans and when we don't understand it. The information could have been communicated through language, learned signals (e.g. traffic signs), or innately recognized signals (e.g. a baby's cry). In other cases, understanding refers to information that was relayed directly through our senses, without the participation of any other human. Whatever the information source may be, it generates in our brain an information structure that has to be compatible with an external information structure. In the case of human communication, the generated structure has to be compatible with an information structure of another person. In the case of direct sensory input, it has to represent in a compatible way a real physical situation. The generated structure consists of concepts that have already existed in our system, and most often, it includes newly formed connections and concepts. The generated structure is activated, thus becoming present in our system. The feeling of understanding or not understanding is an outcome of the analysis that our system performs on that generated information structure.

A communicated information structure consists of primary and secondary information. Primary information is communicated explicitly by the source, and is represented by corresponding firing nodes at the receiver's system. Usually, the primary information invokes in the system secondary information, in the form of additional firing nodes and modifications of connections. Such processes occur automatically in the receiver's system. Secondary firing nodes may be invokes in a variety of situations. For example, primary nodes may cause the activation of detectors, which fire when they detect relationships that exist between concepts that involve the communicated information. Requests to retrieve information may be invoked too by the primary information, as well as instructions to activate projectors and motor units. In addition, firing nodes may invoke changes in the connectivity of the network including forming new connections and modulating the strengths of existing ones. Consequently, secondary nodes that represent classes and wholes become associated with primary nodes and with other secondary nodes, thus fusing the communicated information into the receiver's system.

In communication between humans, the source intends to create a duplicate of a part of its own information structure in the receiver's system. If, as judged by the behavior of the receiver, that has happened, the source assumes that the receiver understood the message. From the other side, the receiver considers the message comprehensible if it did not contain retrieval requests that ended up unanswered or ambiguous, and if no conflicts were generated by it. Conflicts arise when received construction-requests recruit nodes and connections that are in conflict with the already existing circuitry of the receiver. In general, there are two kinds of understanding: subjective and objective. In **subjective understanding**, the receiver's system has not detected any conflicts, ambiguities, or deficiencies in the communicated information structure. In **objective understanding**, the communicated data structure of the receiver matches the data structure of the source–be it another human or a natural situation. Subjective and objective understanding are not always equivalent to each other. A fish that swallowed a bait may have had subjective understanding about the situation, but, alas, not enough objective understanding.

A receiver may misinterpret a message, even if the primary information structures are identical in the sender's and the receiver's systems. The reason is that there might be differences in the rest of their information structures. Usually, the sender and the receiver have had different experiences. If the message calls for relying on such experiences, unexpected receiver's actions may be perceived by the sender as misunderstanding the message. The sender's and the receiver's systems may differ also in the information that they record explicitly and the information that they record implicitly. Explicit information is readily available in processes that rely on retrieval, while implicit information needs to be explicated before it could be used. If implicit information is not explicated, the outcomes of the same process in the two systems may be different.

A communicated information structure may serve as the starting point to internal processes that elaborate on it. These processes, which add new constructors and information retrievers to the original message, may result in uncovering ambiguities and inconsistencies in the elaborated information structure. In such cases, we say that thinking about the message, which was clear at the beginning, has raised questions about its comprehensibility.

Most often, a source would communicate only parts of the information explicitly–the rest has to be completed by the receiver's system. Consequently, there are various levels of understanding, depending on the amount of overlap between the actual information structure of the source and the resulting structure in the receiver's system.

Levels of understanding

Subjective understanding is a basic concept of the system, and it has its own detecting circuitry. In deriving the conclusion about the comprehensibility of a communicated message or a sensed situation, the receiver's system relies on its standard conflict detectors and on indications from its standard data retrieval circuitry. All these signals provide the input to an understanding detector, which checks if its input information contains conflicts, retrieval requests that cannot be met, or retrieval requests that produce ambiguous outcomes. If none of that has happened, the information structure is considered comprehensible. Otherwise, it is considered incomprehensible, and the problematic parts may be highlighted by the understanding-detector, so that they could be further addressed by the system.

Sometimes, we feel that we understand a certain topic better than we understand another one, although we feel that we understand both of them. The depth of our understanding depends on how fused with the rest of our system is the information structure of the topic. Fusion is accomplished by recruiting nodes to represent new concepts and establishing class-exemplar and whole-part connections between nodes. The following example illustrates how understanding increases as communicated information is fused into the existing information structure. Imagine that Einstein meets Archimedes, and after exchanging pleasantries, he decides to explain some highlights from his theory of relativity.

-   E. After some thought-experiments that I performed in my mind, I concluded that mass can be converted into energy.
-   A. I see. Mass can be converted into energy. The same as ice can be converted into water. But what is mass?
-   E. Mass is a property that every object has. The more mass an object has, the harder it is to push it.
-   A. So, it's like weight. We can say that objects have all kinds of properties, one of which is mass. Mass is like a part of an item. And what is energy?

- E. Energy is also a property that some objects have. Objects that have energy can cause other objects to move faster, to move higher, or to be dragged.
- A. So, objects that have energy form a class. For example, wind is an exemplar of that class because wind can drive ships. A drawn bow is another exemplar because it can shoot an arrow to the sky. I guess that Assie should also belong to that class.
- E. What is Assie?
- A. That's my donkey. It can pull the plow, and usually it drags its feet.
- E. Right.
- A. Oh, now I see what you mean. The other day, Assie ate a lot of hay. The mass of the hay disappeared in his body and was converted into energy. He then ran like crazy in the meadow, and then uphill. Luckily, I had energy too, so I ran after him, caught him and dragged him back.
- E. More or less.
- A. What do you mean?
- E. That hay business. Assie ate a lot of hay, all right, but the hay did not loose its mass. It just reappeared a while later in a different form.
- A. Are you sure that the hay did not loose mass in the process?
- E. Trust me.
- A. Fine. Unless you show me an example of an object that looses mass and converts it into energy, forgive me, but your theory is just a pie in the sky.
- E. The sun looses mass to create energy in the form of light, which makes all life possible.
- A. That's beautiful. That's divine.

At this point, "Archimedes" feels that he understands the communicated information. He identified in it the new concepts and the connections between them, and he connected individual concepts and the communicated message as a whole to his own information structure. However, he did not check all the possible connections between the communicated information and his own. Had he done so, he might have pressed more to clarify the concept of mass. That would have given "Einstein" the chance to explain Newton's laws. "Archimedes" would then fuse that information structure into his system, and understand it too.

The understanding process

A lingual message is pre-processed by the system and it is then represented as an information structure that consists of both name-nodes and nodes that represent real experiences (figure 5.12). A pure sensory message is also pre-processed and its representation may also include both name-nodes and real experience nodes. The proportion of name-nodes in the final representation of a message depends on a number of factors such as the contents of the message and the weights of the connections between its name-nodes and their corresponding real-experience-nodes. Both kinds of nodes participate in the process of understanding the message.

The process of understanding a message involves establishing exemplar-class relationships between elements of the message and concepts that make up the system's information structure. The system first tries to match the entire message as an exemplar to one of its concepts. It then tries to relate parts of that message as exemplars to other available concepts. The system may define new items in the message, and then relate them to existing class nodes. A communicated message that develops such connections without raising any feelings of conflicts or ambiguities is considered comprehensible. The more exemplar-class relationships are established between elements of the message and concepts of the system, the deeper is the system's understanding of that message. Usually, the system does not establish all those possible connections. Nevertheless, it can still feel that it understands the message.

In order to understand lingual communication, the system has to establish exemplar-class relationships between the communicated words and nodes that represent lingual concepts. The latter have connections to nodes that represent internal representations of the corresponding experiences (figure 5.12). When those connections are utilized, the communicated message becomes related to internal representations. This enables the formation of more connections between the nodes of the message and nodes of internal representations, thus increasing the understanding of the message. There are many ways in which such connections may be established. Here is one example.

Consider the message 'Joe missed the bus'. The words 'Joe', 'missed' and 'the bus' are name-nodes (figure 5.12). Their corresponding memory record nodes are activated first, and serve as input nodes to the operation sub-unit that interprets the message. The primary goal of this sub-unit is to search the memory and to retrieve a memory record that exactly matches the given phrase. That would mean that the incoming message has been previously encountered by the system. If such a record cannot be found, the message is new, and the next thing would be to retrieve a record whose nodes are classes of the nodes of the message. If 'Joe missed the bus' is not a memory record, the record 'person missed a bus' might be the next best thing, because 'person' is a class node of 'Joe'. The message 'Joe missed the bus' would then be understood as an exemplar of 'person missed a bus'. If the latter record does not exist, the record 'person missed a vehicle' will do. If that record does not exist either, but the record 'Joan missed the train' exists, an operation sub-unit might create from it a generalized record 'person missed a vehicle', and match it with the given phrase. The statement "Joe missed the bus' would then be understood through its analog 'Joan missed the train'.

The phrase 'Joe missed the bus' could be understood also through its projection in various arenas. The projection would consist of a blob that represents Joe and a blob that represents the bus. These blobs would be used in a temporal animation of the process of missing a bus. When such a representation is formed, the suggestion 'Joe missed the bus, and he sat in the back seat of that bus' would trigger the 'incomprehensible' flag. A conflict detector will detect that the blob of Joe has to be projected at two different spots at the same time, which is a basic conflict. This rejection of the second phrase is an indication that the original message has been understood. It resulted from using projectors to simulate the lingual message.

The system will declare a message as incomprehensible in a number of cases. The clearest case is when a conflict is invoked while establishing the representation of the message. Conflicts occur when the message attempts to establish a connection against existing information. For example, if the statement 'Joe eats the bus' is suggested as an exemplar of 'person eats food', 'bus' becomes an exemplar of 'food' while it is also an exemplar of 'not food'. This is a conflict, detectable by conflict detectors. Another major group of incomprehensible messages are those that conflict the grammatical rules of the language. These rules can be expressed as formulas that specify class affiliations of the variables that are substituted into slots. For example, the variable of slot A has to be a verb. If an attempt is made to substitute a noun in slot A, an incomprehensible flag would be raised. Another type of incomprehensible messages are those that do not have enough connections with the rest of the system. For example, 'orthogonal functions are contingent'.

Implications of communicated messages

A communicated message from a source may be understood in different ways by different receivers, due to differences in the background information, which is present in their systems. Such background information may be represented in the system by other co-firing nodes, by primed nodes, or by circuitry that is characteristic to the individual. Primed nodes are nodes that are partially activated to a sub-threshold level. When they receive additional signals from the communicated message, they may start firing and represent the presence of new concepts in the scene. Individual circuitry includes memory records, detectors, and projectors that were acquired through individual experiences. When activated by a message, their response would reflect the individual's experiences. The message 'Joe missed the bus' would be comprehensible to both the parents of Joe and to a stranger: The representation of that message in the stranger's system would include nodes that represent a scene in which a person arrives at a bus stop after the bus has left. In addition, the systems of Joe's parents would have nodes that represent their knowledge about why Joe wanted to take the bus, what Joe is capable of doing if he misses the bus, etc. That circuitry would incorporate the communicated message and create conclusions, represented by firing nodes, such as 'Joe will be late', or 'Joe will get a cab', etc.

Quite often, a source does not spell out explicitly all the information that it intends to convey. Rather, it relays some key elements, based on which the receiver should be able to grasp the entire information structure. The receiver's system carries out standard operations, such as detection, in order to fully understand the situation. These operations uncover and record relationships that exist within the communicated message, and between the communicated message and the rest of the system. The receiver's system also fills-in missing parts, and links the message to the rest of the system, so that it would be accessible in future data retrievals and other operations. For example, a communicated message may contain features that are parts of an item, but the item itself may not be included in the message. The receiver's system, utilizing its detectors and completion mechanisms, can uncover these relationships, recruit a node to represent the missing item, and establish the appropriate connections. Similarly, the receiver's system, using its detectors, can classify items that are not explicitly classified in the message, and assign them as exemplars to existing class nodes. As exemplars, these communicated nodes would inherit properties that reflect experiences of the receiver. Completion processes complete the representation of items that were described in the message only by some of their parts. Overall, the receiver's system, using its circuitry, analyzes the message and incorporates it into the existing circuitry. At the utmost, all the nodes and connections that are implied by a communicated message would be uncovered or formed. Usually, a receiver's system would employ only some of its available mechanisms to uncover the implication of a communicated message or a situation. The more implications are uncovered the deeper is the understanding.

Teachers want their students to develop deep understanding of the learned material. After the first presentation of the material, an initial information structure is developed in the student's system. Repeating the same information may add additional nodes and connections to the initial structure, because some of the communicated information could have been omitted due to various reasons. Then, teachers usually discuss the material and ask questions about it. By participating in these processes, the student's system parses the communicated material and exposes it to various detectors, thus fusion of it with the rest of the system is facilitated, and deeper understanding is achieved.

The discussions in this section illustrated that the feeling of understanding a novel information structure depends on its fusion with the rest of the system. In other words, understanding depends on relationships between the pertinent information structure and a reference structure. The question is what is required of such a reference structure? It seems that the answer would be that any information structure–innate or acquired–that the system understands can serve as a reference. All that is required of such a reference is that it does not invoke any sensation of conflict, ambiguity, or missing elements.

6.   THE MODEL AND THE SIMULATION PROGRAM

In a utopian brain model, each neuron and its synapses would be represented by a node and its connections, and each physiological process would be formulated as a routine. The operation of the model would be coordinated by a simulation program, which would call the appropriate physiological routines at the appropriate time, and figure out their influence on the state of affected nodes. The program would then be able to correlate between the states of the nodes and the macroscopic observed behaviors of the entire system.

In the model presented here, nodes and their connections represent stored information, similar to what is believed to be happening in the brain. Propagation of signals between the nodes is also similar to propagation of activation between neurons. In addition, nodes have parts, which do not have neuronal counterparts. These parts allow the simulation program to affect the state of the nodes without dealing with the physiological mechanisms that cause similar effects in the brain. The simulation program, in effect, integrates many complex physiological mechanisms into pragmatic "bottom line" operations, the details of which are beyond the scope of the model. Such an approach is necessary because of the large number of neurons, the complexity of the system, and the significant gaps in our knowledge of the system.

Nodes have some similarities to neurons, but, in general, each node represents processes that in the real brain are carried out by whole networks of neurons or by parts of a neuron. In the model presented here, nodes can be in a firing state or in a quiet state. Nodes are connected to other nodes by synaptic weights. Activation propagates from firing nodes to the nodes connected to them. These are the main similarities between nodes of the model and real neurons.

In simulating the operation of the brain, the simulation program employs two major groups of routines. The first group is responsible for the proper propagation of signals from a firing node to nodes connected to it. The responsibility of the second group of routines is to modify the connectivity of the network based on the ongoing activities in the firing nodes. The various routines express the operation rules of the system—what might be called the "physiology" of the system. In addition to those two groups of routines, the simulation program has also an "interface" with the external world. This interface sets the initial conditions of the nodes in accordance with the real-life simulated situation, and interprets the outcomes of the simulations vis-a-vis the real-life situation.

To facilitate the operation of the simulation program, nodes and their parts may have numerical attributes with no biological counterparts, such as serial numbers. However, such attributes are used only for "book-keeping" purposes. The model has three types of inter-connected nodes: information nodes, control nodes, and computation units. The information nodes form the information network. The flow of activation in the information nodes simulates the somatic and mental activities that are carried out by the brain. The control nodes simulate the processes that are involved in controlling and coordinating the information flow in the information network. Computation units simulate neural activities that depend on circuitries whose details are beyond the scope of the model. These activities are executed numerically by the simulation program, without any network correlates. Computation units interact with the other nodes through synapses, like regular nodes. Computation units may be of the information or the control types.

The Model

The model can be implemented as a computer simulation program, which consists of two major parts: the interface and the main program. The interface sets the initial state of the networks according to external specification. It then transfer control to the main program, which carries out the actual simulation. Then, control is transferred back to the interface, which interprets the state of the network. Because of the multitude of details that are involved, even with this kind of simulation, the various nodes and their handling by the main program will be outlined first. Then, the components of the nodes will be detailed, and finally, the principles of translating between model representations and external situations will be outlined.

The nodes

Activation of nodes and neurons

The firing of a neuron sends the rest of the system several messages. The sheer firing of the neuron sends the message "I am present in the current situation". On top of that, the pattern of the firing may encode additional information, depending on the neuron and the situation. For example, the frequency of a pulse-train emitted by a pressure sensor encodes the magnitude of the sensed pressure. Firing patterns of other neurons may encode different information, according to the situation.

Once a neuron starts to fire, the duration of its firing depends on the its physiological characteristics. While firing, it may also receive input signals from other neurons, and those inputs may affect the ongoing firing activity.

All these features have to be addressed by the nodes of the model. The main message–I am present–is addressed by the binary nature of the nodes. A node can be in one of two states in accordance with its firing status.

Temporal firing patterns of single neurons are addressed by the model in two ways. First, when different patterns represent different aspects of the same property, such as different magnitudes of the sensed pressure, the neuron would be represented by a group of binary nodes. Each of those nodes represents a different range of the common property, and they are all exemplars of a class-node that represents the general property (e.g. pressure). Second, the model supports explicit temporal patterns that represent other kinds of properties, such as a node being a member of a certain group of active nodes. These patterns are super-imposed numerically by the simulation program on the 'ON' signal of the node. The 'ON' signal serves as the carrier of those supper-imposed patterns. The carrier and the temporal pattern reach all the target nodes that are reached by the 'ON' signal itself. Their effects on the target nodes are calculated by the simulation program. The details of theses processes are elaborated in the following sections.

The duration of the 'ON' state is a parameter of each node, and it can be adjusted to fit the simulated situation. How incoming signals affect an already ongoing firing of a target node is determined by routines of the simulation program, which are tailored to accommodate the specific situation.

Information nodes

Information nodes are responsible for representing all the concepts that can be handled by the model. Figure 6.1 illustrates an information node and its parts. The main part of the information node is its core. Bi-directional

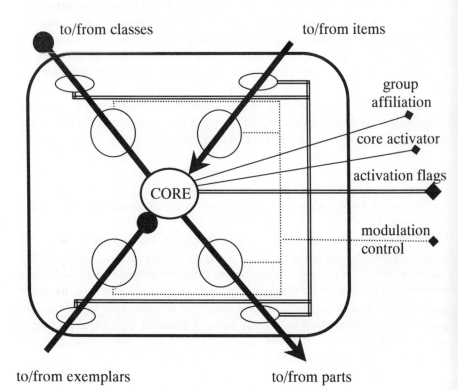

Figure 6.1: The inner structure of a node and the bundles that connect it to the outside. The core of the node integrates the signals arriving through the data-flow bundles and fires if the firing threshold is passed. Each node has a group of control hoop-ups, which can be latched dynamically onto a control unit. These hook-ups include the group affiliation cord, the four bundles that relay source and target firing information, and the four bundles that relay instructions that control the modulators.

Legend: The four circles indicate modulators. The four small ellipses indicate 'flags', which are sensors that provide information about the firing status of target nodes. Thick arrow lines indicate data-flow bundles. All other lines indicate various control bundles.

connections, organized in four bundles, connect a core with cores of other information nodes. A bi-directional connection between two cores consists of two one-directional connections of opposite directionality. Each connection has its own synaptic weight. Each core has a potential that may change with time, and a fixed threshold (default value of one). When the core's potential is greater than the threshold, the core fires. A firing core sends unit signals through all its enabled outgoing connections. The simulation program may super-impose temporal patterns on this unit signal.

The potential of the core at an arbitrary time t, $P_i(t)$, is given by formula [6.1].

$$P_i(t) = f\left(P_i(t - \Delta t), \sum_j M_j \cdot \sigma_{ji} \cdot I_j\right) \qquad [6.1]$$

$P_i(t)$ depends on the potential at the previous time interval, $P_i(t - \Delta t)$, and on the weighted sum of the signals that have arrived during the previous time interval, $\sum_j M_j \cdot \sigma_{ji} \cdot I_j$. The function that specifies the exact form of that dependency, f, matches the simulated situation. The index i indicates the receiving node, j are indices of sending nodes, σ_{ji} are synaptic weights from nodes j to node i, M_j is the modulation factor of σ_{ji}, and I_j is the intensity of the signal sent by node j. The intensity I_j may have two components. The first is the carrier signal, which is one if node j is firing and zero if it is quiet. The second component is the temporal pattern, which is super-imposed on the carrier. The second component can be expressed as an array of numbers or as a function.

The simulation program can employ special routines to evaluate the effects of the second components of the I_j's on the core potential of the receiving node i. Here are few examples. In the simplest case, the carriers of all incoming signals are integrated regardless of their superimposed patterns. All the one-components of the I_j in [6.1], and only them, are considered in the summation. In a second case, only the ones of I_j's that carry a specific super-imposed pattern are added. This way, only contribution from a specified group of firing nodes affect node j. Contributions from nodes that don't have the matching pattern or from those that don't have a pattern at all are ignored. In general, matches between patterns can be used to add terms that are non-linear in the I_j's to the sigma of equation [6.1].

The simulation program can decide which of the incoming super-imposed patterns will be relayed from node i to other nodes, and super-impose them on the output signals on node i.

The cores represent the concepts of the system. Firing cores represent the current state of the system: what it senses, what it feels, and what it is doing.

The four bundles of each core represent the four fundamental relationships between concepts: part-item, item-part, exemplar-class, and class-exemplar. These are encoded by the synaptic weights of the corresponding one-directional connections (as detailed in chapter 2).

In addition to the core and the four bundles, which represent the information stored by the system, nodes have parts whose main purpose is to facilitate the use of the stored information in thinking and other processes. These parts are responsible for detecting and controlling certain aspects of the function of the core. They include modulation controllers, firing flags, group affiliation detectors, and core activators. These parts are organized in control bundles, and they relay their information between nodes that represent data and control units that control data-flow in the system.

Each of the four modulation-control bundles conveys instruction for setting the modulation factors of its bundle. These instructions can slightly increase or decrease the modulation factor, completely block the bundle, or set the factor to maximum value. Modulation factors can also be used to superimpose a **label** on outgoing signals that pass through the bundle. Modulation is an important element in the operation of thinking units.

Firing flags convey information about the firing status of the core itself and of downstream nodes. Based on the latter information, a thinking unit can evaluate the effects of its manipulation of the modulators. It can determine if the activity of downstream nodes remained the same, increased, or decreased right after changing a modulation factor. Firing flags also help in the identification of the end products of retrieval processes. End products are such nodes that are being activated by the request, but do not participate in the activation of other nodes. An end product of a retrieval process does not participate in the activation of other nodes.

The group affiliation bundle conveys information about labels that are superimposed on the firing core. This information enables other units to consider or to ignore a firing node in their computations. The group affiliation bundle also conveys information if the core is commissioned or not. A non-commissioned node can be recruited to represent new information, while a commissioned node can only be updated with certain relevant information.

The core-activator activates the core node upon the request of a thinking unit. It can maintain this activity for as long as the thinking unit requests. The thinking unit can label the activated core through the core activator. The label is a small temporal activation pattern that is super-imposed on the ON output signal of the firing core. This label propagates to all the nodes that receive signals from the firing core. If those nodes surpass their threshold, the label will be super-imposed also on their output. This label provides identification to the downstream activated-cores, so that they could be recognized by other parts of the system.

Control nodes and control units

The control channels of information-nodes are handled by fundamental control units. A **fundamental control unit** consists of control-nodes, which do not represent concepts of the system. Their responsibility is to handle the various control elements of the information-node to which they are connected. A fundamental control unit may be connected permanently to the control channels of one information-node, or it may have hook-ups that can be connected temporarily to different information-nodes, according to the needs of the system. The control-nodes of a fundamental control unit are either activators or sensors of sub-units of the information-node that they control. Like information nodes, control nodes are activated according to formula [6.1] by input signals received from other nodes.

Activator nodes, which are included in a fundamental control unit, are: a node that causes the core of the controlled information-node to fire; a node that inhibits the core from firing; nodes that increase the modulation factor of the controlled bundle (one per bundle); and nodes that decreases the modulation factor of a bundle (one per bundle).

The sensor-nodes of the fundamental control unit are: a node that detects the firing of the core; a node that detects the label of the firing core; nodes that detect the status of the flags (one node per bundle); and a node that detects if the core is commissioned or is it available for recruitment.

Construction units and the long distance network

Construction units modify synaptic weights between nodes. This includes forming new synapses, increasing or decreasing weights of existing synapses, and eliminating synapses. Each of these operations is executed by a corresponding construction unit. The specific construction unit is triggered by the node that requests the modification. The nodes whose synapses have to be modified have first to be marked. The construction unit then effectuates the requested changes. The construction unit need not be physically connected only to the affected nodes. It may broadcast its instruction to the entire system, but only the marked nodes would be tuned to this broadcast and respond by carrying out the requested construction.

It may happen that two nodes, which are not connected, need to establish a new connection. If these nodes are further apart from each other, they may have to rely on the long distance network in forming the connection. The long distance network facilitates the formation of connections between distant nodes. The request to establish a long distance connection is issued by an ongoing operation of the system. Such a request has to identify the nodes that need to be connected, and the type of connection. The involved nodes may be identified by labeling them, e.g. by superimposing a temporal firing pattern on their outgoing signals. Once they have been identified, they hook-up to the long distance network. The long distance network provides a channel that connects these nodes. This channel is then used to establish the requested synaptic weight between the nodes. The simulation program modifies connections based on signals that it receives from construction units, and based on the corresponding label signals, which are emitted by the marked nodes.

New connections may be made between any type of nodes–information nodes or control nodes. Making new connections or modifying existing ones between information-nodes changes the information contents of the system. Making such changes between control-nodes and information-nodes provides flexibility in processing the existing information. It makes it possible for the circuitry of a thinking unit to perform thinking activities on various node populations.

Computation units

While it is assumed that all data processing in the brain is done by its neural circuitry, the simulation model will allow the participation of outside processors in various data processing tasks. Outside processors are routines of the simulation program that process information for the simulation model. The reason for relying on outside processors is that many brain processes are known only by their input and output, but not by their detailed circuitry. For example, the brain can classify events by the order of their temporal occurrence. It is not known (at least at this time) what brain circuitry is involved in such determinations. If the simulation model needs to analyze temporal ordering of events, the necessary analysis would be done by outside processors. Another example is our ability to recognize circles when we see them. It is not known what circuitry in the brain recognizes circles and analyzes them. Therefore, information about circles in the field of view would be provided in the simulation by outside processors. The system could incorporate the provided information in its own operations.

A **computation unit** is a processing element that exchanges information with the nodes of the model, but processes the information on its own. Computation units may contain circuitry of regular nodes, but they may also rely on computations done by outside processors. All the regular nodes process information according to the same rules, as outlined above [6.1], while each computation unit may have its own rules of processing information. However, nodes and computation-units communicate with each other like nodes. They encode information as patterns of active nodes, and the activation of computation units is triggered by signals from other nodes.

As an example of a computation unit, consider classifiers. Classifiers can be found in various modules, and each arena has many of them. From practical reasons, some simulation programs may consider classification to be a fundamental process, the details of which are of no interest to the task at hand. In such cases, classifiers may be represented as computation units. The following is an illustration of processes, which are done by the nodes of a classification unit, transparent to the main simulation program.

A classifier does two main operations: First, it detects certain required features in the incoming information flow. These features would make an item eligible to become an exemplar of the class associated with the detector. Then, the classifier establishes the exemplar-class relationships between the item and the class.

The detector is triggered when a group of active nodes contains a certain pattern. That activated pattern makes the entire group eligible to become an exemplar of the class to which the detector is pointing. For example, a motion detector in the visual field may be triggered by a pattern of 'moving' pixels, which are parts of an object. The entire object becomes an exemplar of a class 'objects that have moving parts'. If this entire group is not yet represented as an item, an item node is recruited to represent it. The item node becomes an exemplar of the class node, as illustrated in the figure 6.2. The processes of detection, recruitment of an item node, and establishing new connections are executed by the simulation program. The simulation program does not rely on neural processes, such as propagation of activation, to bring about these changes in the network.

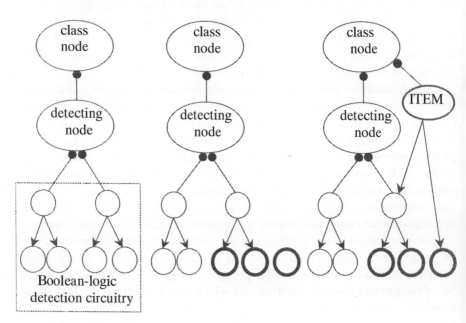

1. THE DETECTOR 2. A GROUP OF ACTIVE 3. THE GROUP OF ACTIV
                      NODES IS DETECTD   NODES IS RECORDED

Figure 6.2: Processes that take place inside a computation unit of a detector.

In detection, the direction of the information flow is from the Boolean-logic detection circuitry to the detector, and from there to the class node. A computation unit that acts as a detector can act also as a projector, if the direction of the information-flow is reversed. The detecting node is activated first. It then activates a selected chain of its exemplars and their parts, down the Boolean-logic circuitry to the input nodes of the detector. For example, if the detector in the figure 6.2 detects moving objects, its detecting node will fire when stimuli from a moving object activate the input nodes of its detection circuitry. This detector acts as a projector when its detecting node is activated by a unit of the system, and signals propagate down to its input nodes and activate them, thus mimicking a moving object.

The Dynamics of the Model

The goal of the connectionist model presented here is to define a system, consisting of nodes and connections, which can simulate a variety of brain activities and situations. In particular, it should be able to simulate mental and somatic processes that happen concurrently in the brain. Nodes represent concepts, and connections between nodes represent relationships between concepts. Patterns of active nodes represent the ongoing activity of the system. Sensory nodes become active by events outside of the system. "Pacemaker nodes" keep firing on their own all the time. The rest or the nodes become active by signals that they receive from other nodes. Some nodes represent computation units. They interact with the rest of the system by sending and receiving signals, but they have their own rules of processing the signals that they receive.

The simulation program coordinates two major activities in the model: propagation of signals in the network, and modification of connections between nodes. Time is divided into discrete intervals. Propagation of signals takes place in even time intervals, and modification of connections occurs in odd time intervals. First, the simulation program sets the initial circuitry and activates nodes that represent the initial state of the system. Formally, activating the nodes that represent the initial state occurs at the zero'th time interval, and the initial setting of the synaptic weights is at the first time interval. Then, the simulation program propagates signals from the firing nodes to nodes connected to them, based on the connections at the first time interval. This is how the core potentials of the nodes at the second time interval are figured out, using equation [6.1]. The program determines which nodes passed the firing threshold at the second time interval. The program treats differently firing information nodes and firing control nodes. Control-nodes that fire at the second time interval express modifications that have to be made to connections between nodes. The simulation program implements these modifications in the third time interval. It then propagates signals from nodes that were firing in the second time interval to nodes connected to them, based on the existing synaptic weights in the third time interval. That is how the state of the nodes in the fourth time interval is obtained. The simulation program keeps propagating signals and updating synapses in this way repeatedly. In addition, the simulation program activates computation units. Since computation units operate at their own pace, the simulation program takes care of synchronizing their interactions with the rest of the system. Information is exchanged between computation units and regular nodes in the appropriate discrete time intervals. Figure 6.3 illustrates the sequence of operations of the simulation program.

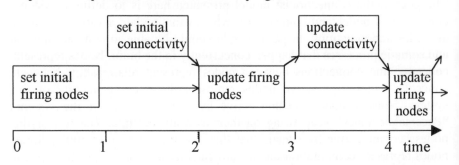

Figure 6.3: The sequence of events that are coordinated by the simulation program.

The simulation program propagates signals relying on the existing connectivity between firing nodes and quiet nodes, as explained above [6.1]. The connections specify to the program to which nodes the signals should propagate. The situation with modification of connections is more complicated. It may be necessary to establish a new connection between unconnected nodes, or to modify an existing connection between nodes. The simulation program needs to rely on some physical means to identify the involved nodes. In the model, each request to modify a connection includes two parts: identifying the involved nodes, and specifying the nature of the modification. A control-unit that requests a modification supplies this information to the simulation program. It identifies the involved nodes by **marking** or **labeling** them. Inducing specific temporal firing patterns is one of the physical means that can be used for marking nodes. The control unit marks the nodes, and supplies those marks to the simulation program, thus enabling the identification of the nodes. In the model, each type of connection modification (e.g. increase synaptic weight, change modulation factor, etc.) has its own node. Firing of that node signifies to the simulation program that the modification has to be executed. The main purpose of using labels is to enable the system to perform concurrently different tasks that involve changes of connections. Should the system be limited to having only one such task at a time, labels may not be so crucial. In biological systems, connections modification processes may be at the sub-neural level. Mechanisms that are not controlled by firing of neurons may cause these changes in biological systems.

The firing state of a node at any time interval can be represented by a binary variable: one for firing and zero for quiet. Some processes, such as labeling, may require greater temporal resolution. In such cases, the even and odd time intervals may be further divided into sub-intervals, the number of which would depend on the required temporal resolution. The analysis of labels would be carried out by the simulation program based on the firing patterns in those temporal-sub-intervals.

In some cases, connections have to be established between unconnected nodes. In other cases, connections between some of the firing nodes have to be modified, while others have to remain unchanged. In all those cases, the program identifies the involved nodes by their labels. The simulation program can modify connections between active nodes that have a common label. The labels themselves are superimposed on the output of nodes in even time-intervals, by signals that propagate via connections from a marking node to the labeled node. In the simulations, labeling relies on connections that explicitly exist in the simulated network. On the other hand, modifications of connections, which take place in odd time intervals, may rely in part on "virtual hardware". The simulation program generates the modification without relying on any supporting network hardware. For example, when the simulation program establishes a synapse between two distant unconnected nodes, it does it based on their common label, as encoded by the activities of the nodes. Recognizing the two common labels and bridging the two nodes are not supported by any network hardware. It is assumed that such hardware exists, but its details are beyond the scope of the simulation program.

The simulation program contains a human-interpretation-interface, which translates human information into network representations and vice versa. The human-interpretation-interface keeps a list of the conceptual meaning of the nodes that the model uses. It can translate relationships between human concepts into synaptic weights between their corresponding nodes, and vice versa.

The building blocks of the simulation program

The system consists of objects that are handled by the main simulation program. The objects are generated from prototypes. There are prototypes for synapses, information nodes, control units, construction units, and computation units. An object will usually have elements that specify its hardware properties, its dynamic states, and operations related to it. Objects perform their own calculations, using embedded routines.

Each object has a unique serial number, which is assigned by the main program. These serial numbers are used by the objects when they interact with each other. However, the main program makes the serial number of one object available to another object based on some physiological justification. For example, in order for node A to establish a synapse with node B, node A would need the serial number of node B. The main program would provide this number to node A only if node B has been labeled with a certain label, and node A can provide to the main program the same label.

The main program operates a "clock", whose ticks are used by the objects to perform and synchronize their activities.

Following are descriptions of the various prototypes and their properties. Objects have their own serial numbers, and they also contain serial numbers of other objects. Those serial numbers are assigned and provided by the main program, when it creates the object according to the prototype or during initiation. The creation of an object is prompted by requests from nodes that provide the necessary "physiological" features.

The synapse

A synapse connects a signal-sending node and a signal-receiving node. The intensity of the sent signal is multiplied by the synaptic weight and integrated by the core of the receiving node, according to formula [6.1]. The elements of a synapse are:

- The value of the synaptic weight.
- Serial number of the node that sends the signals.
- Serial number of the node that receives the signals.
- The serial number of the bundle to which the synapse belongs.
- A delay element.
- A synapse can be defined initially in the first time interval or in a subsequent odd time intervals (figure 6.3) by a request from

construction units. Modifications of a synaptic weight or disconnecting a synapse are also requested by construction units in odd time intervals.

The delay element is a parameter that specifies the time delay between sending the signal and its arrival to the target node. If the simulation is not concerned with this feature, the delay remains at its default value–zero. Otherwise, it is set according to the needs when the synapse is defined.

The information of a synapse is used by the nodes that it connects, to propagate signals according to formula [6.1].

The information node

Information nodes form networks that encode and represent information. A firing information node indicates the presence of its represented entity in the current scene. Some information nodes have a lingual meaning. The main program keeps these meanings on file, and utilizes them in the process of translating from lingual to nodal representation, and vice versa. (More about this subject can be found in the next section). An information node has the following elements:

- Connections with other nodes: A connection consists of a pair of synapses with opposite polarities. The information node has a list of all the serial numbers of its synapses. The list is divided into four sub-lists, for the four data bundles of the node: part to item, item to part, exemplar to class, and class to exemplar. Each of these sub-lists is divided to two: one for outgoing synapses, and the other for incoming ones. A node may have connections in all its bundles, only in some of them, or no connection at all (un-assigned node). When a connection is added to a node, the main program updates all the serial numbers related to the node and its bundle.
- Serial number of each bundle.
- An array of four elements, one per bundle, that stores the current value of the modulation factor of its bundle. A modulation factor modulates all the outgoing signals through its bundle by the same factor (according to formula [6.1]). Modulation factors are set in initiation or by requests from control nodes, in odd time intervals.
- An array of four elements, one per bundle, that stores flag information. The flag indicates the number of downstream nodes that were activated in whole or in part by the node. The control flags are

set by the main program in even time intervals, based on the activities of the relevant nodes.

- Firing indicator. A binary variable that indicates if the node is firing (1) or quiet (0). The firing indicator is regulated by an internal routine of the node.

- Firing counter. This counter is responsible for shutting-off the firing of the node after a prescribed number of time intervals that have elapsed from the onset of its firing, or from the arrival of the last input signal. The firing-duration time is defined for each node based on the simulated situation. The firing counter is regulated by an internal routine in accordance with time information from the main program.

- Commission indicator. A binary variable that indicates if the node is already recruited (1) or is it unassigned (0). This indicator is regulated by an internal routine, and is updated in odd time intervals, based on the changes in the connectivity of the node.

- Time-tick receiver. This element facilitates the synchronization of the activities of the node with the external clock. It provides the time index t that is used by the core-integrator. This variable is provided by the main program.

- Core–integrator. This element receives the incoming signals and generates the output potential of the node according to formula [6.1]. It separates between the carrier of each signal and the temporal pattern, which is super-imposed on the carrier. It uses this information to update the output carrier and the labels of the node. In determining the core's potential and the output of the node, the core integrator also considers signals received through the core activator and the group affiliation hook-ups.

Marker nodes

Marker nodes are control nodes, and they operate as parts of larger control and construction units. They are connected to the control hook-ups of information nodes, through which they relay labeling signals. Those labels mark the receiving nodes for further manipulations, such as adjustments of modulation factors or modifying or adding connections. Connections between labeled nodes can be added or modified according to instructions that are broadcast from connection-construction nodes. The broadcasts are sent to a large population of receiving nodes, but only the labeled ones are affected. A marker-node can label the core of a labeled node, or any of its data bundles. Labeling a core is done by superimposing a small temporal pattern on the core potential. All the outgoing signals of the labeled node will carry the label of the core with them to downstream nodes, which will become labeled too. When a marker-node labels only a data bundle, only downstream nodes will become labeled. This type of labeling is used when a variable node, which is connected to a slot node of a computation unit, has to be labeled by that unit. Only the variable node, and not the slot node, has to be marked for further manipulation. In addition to identifying the node, the label may include an indication whether the labeled node is the receiving node and/or the sending node of the connection to be established. One marker-node can label both receiving and sending nodes.

The elements of marker-nodes are:

- Firing indicator.
- The type of the marker. (A marker of cores or bundles)
- The temporal pattern of the label. This pattern is superimposed on the receiving nodes. In practice, recognizing labels by network mechanisms that analyze temporal patterns is beyond the scope of the simulation program. Instead, the label would be represented by a number, unique to its issuing node. The simulation program relays this number to the appropriate receiving nodes, which store it. These numbers are used in the next odd time-interval by the simulation program to identify nodes whose connections should be modified.
- A bundle of output connections. Each output connection relays the label of the marker-node to a receiving node. It also relays a code indicating the role of the receiving node in the intended change, e.g. a new exemplar in exemplar to class connection, or increase existing part-to-item synaptic weight. Each output connection contains the serial number of the receiving node and the code of its role in the change. This information is passed to the marker node by the control unit or the construction unit to which it belongs.

Some examples of incorporating marker-nodes in a variety of computation units will be given in the next chapter.

Connection-construction node

These are also control nodes. When firing, a connection-construction node causes the execution of all the pending connection-modification-requests in a group of subordinate nodes. This group may include only localized nodes, or it may cover the entire system. These nodes have been labeled by marker nodes, as explained above. The elements of a connection-construction-node are:

- Firing indicator.
- The serial numbers of the nodes that are under the control of the connection-construction node. This list if relayed to the main program, and with information already received there about the labels of the nodes to be modified, the main program updates the appropriate connections.

The modulation control unit

The unit consists of modulation control nodes that when fired cause changes in the modulators of their subordinate information nodes. The elements of a modulation control unit are:

- The serial numbers of subordinate nodes.
- Arrays of four nodes, one per bundle, that control the following activities: increasing a modulation factor by a set amount, decreasing a modulation factor by a certain amount, and inhibiting the bundle. These activities are mutually exclusive to each other in the same bundle.

Flags-sensors unit

The flags-sensors unit contains flag-sensor nodes, which are control nodes. These nodes fire in accordance with the status of the flags of their controlled information-node. Flags sense the induced activity, or lack thereof, in nodes that receive signals from the controlled information-node. They are parts of the information-node, and they are being updated by the main program. Their main importance is in the evaluation of the outcome of retrieval requests. Flag-sensor nodes relay this information to other computation units. The elements of each node are:

- Serial number of the controlled node.

- An array of four nodes, one per bundle, that indicate the status of the corresponding flag in the controlled information-node.

Core labeling and activation sensor

This control node senses the activation status and picks-up the label or labels of the core of its controlled information-node. This information is made available to the computation unit to which this core-labeling-and-activation sensor belongs. The elements of this sensor node are:

- Firing indicator.
- Label or labels that the sensor picks-up.
- Serial number of subordinate node.

Computation units

Computation units are represented as special nodes that communicate with the rest of the system through regular connections, but perform their computations according to their own rules and scheduling. Control units, connection-construction units, and retrieval units are examples of computation units. A computation unit will usually contain regular nodes and non-nodal elements that perform some of the computation. The main program is actually responsible for executing these computations and coordinating the information exchange with the rest of the system. The interface of a computation unit with the rest of the system, through which information between the two is exchanged, consists of elements that behave like regular nodes. The system has various prototypes of computation units, based on which computation-unit objects are formed. The elements of a computation unit are:

- Input slots. An input slot is an interface node that can be connected to nodes outside of the computation unit. Those outside nodes can be called 'variable nodes'. When the connection happens, we say that the variable node fills the slot, or is latched to the slot. For a variable node to fill a slot, both nodes have first to be labeled. Then, the appropriate connections between them are established. Each slot has one or more marker nodes. When triggered, they label the slot and the variable node that has to fill it. This leads to the formation of the necessary connections between the variable node and the computation unit. Such a marker has a permanent connection to its slot. In addition, all the system-nodes that might possibly fill the slot are connected or can be connected to the marker. When the marker fires, it triggers and labels the slot, and at the same time, it labels firing system-nodes that are connected to it. This marking utilizes permanent or temporary connections that exist between the marker and the variable nodes. A connection-construction node can then establish the necessary connection between the variable node and the slot-node.

- Output slots. These are similar to input slots, but the variable nodes that fill them are outputs of the computation program, instead of inputs. Like an input slot, an output slot has associated marker nodes that mark the output variable node, and enable the formation of the connection between the slot and its variable.

- Shared nodes. These nodes of the computation unit are also regular nodes of the external system.

- Computation program. This is the routine that performs the intended activities of the computation unit.

- Program initiation node. When fired, this interface node triggers the actual execution of the unit's computation program. The organization of the computation unit is such that the program starts its computations only after its input slots have been filled.

- Done node. The firing of this node indicates to the system that the program finished its computation. The main program relies on such information when it coordinates activities of many objects.

- Shut-off node. Activation of this node terminates all activities of the unit. This node can be activated internally, when all the steps of the computation have been finished, or externally, when the computations have to stop before reaching its normal end.

The Language Interface (brain reading)

In the simulation process, patterns of active nodes represent patterns of active neurons in the brain. The latter are directly related to states of activity of the body, to sensations and feelings that the body experiences, and to states of mind. On the other hand, those states of the body and the mind can be described by human language. Hence, expressions in human language are correlated with underlying activation patterns of nodes. The simulation program has a language interface that can translate an internal representations of activated patterns of nodes into their corresponding lingual expressions (a word, a phrase, or a group of sentences), and vice versa.

Words are assembled into sentences according to grammatical rules of human languages, so that complex situations can be described by fundamental concepts. Similarly, simple patterns of activated nodes, which correspond to fundamental concepts, are assembled into complex patterns that describe situations that are more complex. "Grammatical" analysis of a pattern of activated nodes describes how the pattern is related to its constituting elements. This analysis specifies several things. First, it specifies which nodes were firing at the relevant time intervals. Second, it specifies which nodes activated which nodes, and third, it specifies which bundles conveyed activation between the participating nodes. The program that translates nodal into lingual expressions relies on this grammatical analysis, and on lexical information, which is permanently associated with each nodal concept. The lexical information is about the meaning of the nodes and their connections.

In the model and in the brain, concepts may be represented by patterns of active nodes (distributed representation). When translating a scene, each of its concepts that is represented in a distributed way has to be identified first, so that its presence could be discerned. The lexicon used in the translation should consist not only of the meaning of single nodes or neurons, but also of the meaning of patterns.

Information-nodes represent atomic and relational concepts of the system. Some nodes have associated names, which are lingual descriptions of the meaning of the nodes (e.g. 'green' means that the firing of the node associated with this name indicates that 'green' is part of the present scene). Nodes that do not have names can be described through their relationships with named nodes. For example, an unnamed node that has been recruited to represent a new flavor can be described as 'a combination of peach and banana flavors', if the nodes that sense the flavors of peach and banana have names.

The name of a node that represents an atomic concept is its direct lingual translation. A node that represents a relational concept has slot nodes, which can be connected to variable patterns. A relational-concept-node fires when patterns that possess certain features activate its slot nodes. The lingual translation of a scene that consists of a relational concept and its variable activators is determined by the names of the involved nodes and their relative roles in the pattern.

As an example, figure 6.4 illustrates how the lingual expression 'the cloud is higher than the mountain' can be extracted from patterns of firing nodes, which were formed when a certain scene, consisting of a cloud and a mountain, stimulated the system.

Visual stimuli of a certain cloud and a certain mountain have entered an arena and recruited nodes to represent them. Those representations were analyzed by the detectors of the arena, which uncovered the relationship that the cloud is higher than the mountain. This conclusion was represented by the firing of the appropriate nodes.

The process of translating the firing pattern of figure 6.4 into a lingual expression is done in steps. First, unnamed nodes get names. Node X, which represents a variable pattern, does not have a name of it own. Since it is an exemplar of the named node 'cloud', it gets the name 'the cloud'. Similarly, node Y gets the name 'the mountain', node x3 gets the name 'the height of the cloud', and node y1 gets the name 'the height of the mountain'. (In the last two expressions, the nodal relationship 'A is a part of B' is translated into the lingual expression 'A of B'.) Then, the names of variable nodes that activate the slot nodes of the relational concept and the name of the relational concept itself are merged. Since node X (the cloud) activates slot A, and node Y (the mountain) activates slot B, their names are substituted in the name of the concept 'A is higher than B'. The resulting lingual expression is 'the cloud is higher than the mountain'.

The type of connection between nodes, which is indicated by the bundle that contains the connection, makes it possible to translate patterns of nodal activation into lingual expression, as illustrated above. Correlating the activation of patterns of real neurons with lingual expression is more complex. One of the reasons is that while the basic relationships class-exemplar and whole-part are embedded in the nodes, they are probably not encoded explicitly in real neurons. Another reason is that the model distinguishes between information nodes and control nodes. At this time, it is not known if all the neurons are information-neurons, and if not, how to distinguish between information and control neurons. Before being able to translate a pattern of firing neurons into a lingual expression, at least two things have to be established. First, that only information neurons are translated. Second, the nature of those basic relationships between the firing information-neurons has to be spelled out. Those relationships depend not

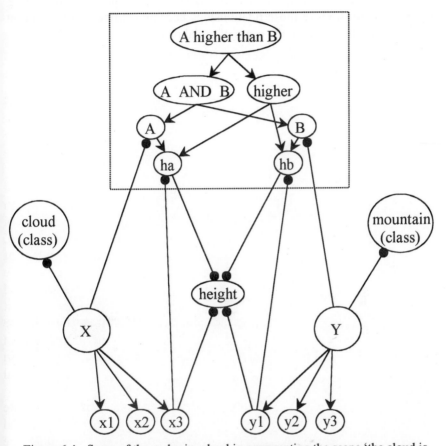

Figure 6.4: Some of the nodes involved in representing the scene 'the cloud is higher than the mountain'. x1, x2, and x3 are properties of a certain cloud X, which is higher than a certain mountain Y, whose properties are y1, y2, and y3. The features x1, x2, and x3 recruited the node X to represent them as an item. A detector, such as in figure 6.2, (not shown here) classified X as a cloud, and made it an exemplar of the class 'cloud'. Similarly, y1, y2, and y3 recruited Y to represent them as an item, which was detected and classified as an exemplar of the class 'mountain'. The height of the cloud (x3) and the height of the mountain (y1) activated the 'higher detector' (in the dotted box) that connected X to slot A, and Y to slot B. Words indicate named nodes, and meaningless letter-combinations indicate unnamed nodes.

only on the firing neurons, but also on the synaptic weights between firing and quiet neurons. Once those relationships become explicit, the translation could proceed much like in the cases of nodal patterns.

7.   THE MACHINERY OF SOME MENTAL PROCESSES

The synaptic weights determine the **flow of activation** from firing nodes to quiet ones. In thinking processes, values of synaptic weights are modulated right before the activation propagates through them from the firing nodes. This stage of modulation of synaptic weights, which is temporary in nature, is what distinguishes flow of activation in general from **thinking processes**. The purpose of the modulation is to direct the flow of activation according to the specifications of the thinking unit. The system can support concurrently thinking processes and non-thinking activation flows. This chapter describes in greater detail the structure of basic circuitries that serve as building blocks to a variety of thinking processes, which were outlined above. The emphasis in these descriptions is on the way that the circuitries interact with the database, utilizing only the fundamental operations, and relying on the fundamental relationships that exist between nodes.

Thinking routines

A thinking routine is a circuitry that has the responsibility of performing a certain thinking task. It has input nodes, inner nodes, and output nodes. The output nodes can activate various patterns of nodes, which do not belong to the routine itself. A thinking routine is triggered by external signals. It then performs its task at its own scheduling and pace. When the task is completed, the routine activates the output pattern, and sends a signal that it is done. The activities of a thinking routine may be terminated by outside units, e.g. if the routine fails to provide an output within a certain time window. Thinking routines form networks, which carry out the thinking processes of the system. Signals that individual thinking routines send out are used in the coordination of their activities. Different thinking routines can function concurrently with each other.

Triggering of a thinking routine is initiated from outside of the routine, beyond its control. Some routines may be able to handle a new triggering when an old one is still being processed, and some won't. In the latter cases, the routine has a mechanism that shuts off its input channels during its operation.

The input nodes of a thinking routine consist of fixed input nodes and of slot nodes. Fixed input nodes are activated by outside nodes with which they have permanent connections. However, various activity patterns of those outside nodes can activate the same fixed input node, depending on the external event. Unlike fixed input nodes, **slots** are activated by outside nodes with which they establish temporary connections. It is said that such outside nodes **latch** onto the slot for the current task, and then they are disconnected when the task is completed. The long distance network enables the latching of outside nodes onto slots. A unit that triggers a thinking routine has to label the intended input nodes, so that they could be latched onto the appropriate slots. Similarly, the output nodes of a thinking routine consist of fixed output nodes and output slots. The thinking routine labels its outcome nodes, so that they could be recognized by other units that need them. Based on its label, it should be possible to identify the process to which the labeled outcome node belongs. Thinking routines that have slots operate as centers for thinking activities that can serve distant node populations. The reach of routines that do not have slots is usually more limited.

Inputs to a thinking routine may be continuing or transient. Transient inputs cease to fire before the thinking routine has completed its task. The system has means to maintain the activation of transient inputs, if their continued activation is needed for the thinking process. In certain cases, a routine may treat the termination of an input signal as a relevant piece of information, which is considered in the thinking process.

Thinking routines may require input of certain characteristics, such as being an exemplar of a certain class. The thinking routine may block inputs that do not satisfy its requirements. The routine may issue a message that an unacceptable input was attempted and was blocked.

Inner nodes of a thinking routine are activated by input nodes and by other inner nodes. The output nodes of the routine are activated by input nodes and by inner nodes. The output of a routine contains information that is the result of the thinking process, and information about the status of the thinking process itself and the nature of the results. For example, in addition to present a solution, a thinking routine may provide information about the degree that the solution satisfies all the requirements of the problem.

In the process of thinking, a routine may activate nodes that have to be used by other routines or by later steps of the routine itself. These nodes must be recognizable by their future users. The mere firing of a node cannot be relied upon as a recognition means, because nodes may be activated by a variety of unrelated concurrent events. The thinking routine needs to be able to label any node that it activates as such, so that it could be recognized by users that rely on it. One possible labeling mechanism would be by superimposing a typical temporal firing pattern on the output signal of the labeled node. The actual superimposing of a label on the outgoing signal can be done by the modulator, which controls the signals of the outgoing bundle of the active node. Units that have to use the labeled node are provided with the temporal 'key' to recognize the label. The labeled node is recognized by the user based on the match between the label and the key. A node that is activated by several thinking routines at the same time would have the labels of all of them. Each user should be able to recognize its own superimposed label in such multi-label firing nodes. Another possible mechanism for identifying a node to a user-unit would be by establishing a common exchange node. The node that the thinking routine needs to provide to another user is connected as an exemplar to the exchange node. The other user is wired to look for an exemplar of the exchange node. The user considers the exemplar of the exchange node as the node that it has to use.

The basic operations that thinking routines perform may be divided into three major categories: activation, detection, and internal processing. Activation operations include issuing retrieval requests to memory units, activating motor units, activating projectors in arenas, activating other thinking routines, activating output nodes, and activating constructors. Detection operations include detecting patterns of external stimuli, detecting situations that are generated in the arenas by projectors and by external stimuli, and detecting retrieved data. Internal operations generate the output of the system from the input that it receives. All of these operations are composed of the fundamental operations: activation of nodes, controlling modulators, establishing connections between nodes, and eliminating connections between nodes. The next sections will illustrate how some common thinking routines can be put together from these fundamental operations.

A fundamental operation, which takes part in a thinking routine, is triggered by a requesting node. The requesting node has to label the variables on which the requested fundamental operation is expected to operate. This must be done because many fundamental operations may be running concurrently, and each one of them has to be operating on its intended variables. If the outcome of a fundamental operation is an activated node that has to be considered by other operations, it should also be labeled. The model discussed here takes labeling for granted, and does not deal with the mechanics of the labeling process. An operation may be required to operate on nodes that are distant from each other. In such cases, the long distance network provides the necessary support for long distance communication. The mechanisms of these processes are also beyond the realm of the model discussed here.

The activation of a thinking routine is initiated by a requesting circuitry. The requesting circuitry has direct contact with the slots and with the trigger node of the thinking routine. If the thinking routine has input slots, the requesting circuitry labels the input variables, thus enabling their latching onto the appropriate input slots of the thinking routine. The requesting circuitry also provides a label to the thinking routine, so that the outcome of the operation could be labeled if needed. When the requesting circuitry completes all these preliminary steps, it activates the trigger node of the thinking routine. Formally, an activation request has the following elements: an optional array of labels that are used to identify the input variables, a direct connection to the node of the circuitry of the thinking routine that launches the operation, and optional labels for the outcome nodes.

Retrieval requests

Retrieval requests constitute an important group of thinking routines. A retrieval request characterizes target nodes based on their specified relationships with other given nodes. The fundamental retrieval requests are those that retrieve nodes that have one of the four fundamental relationships (exemplar, class, part, or item) with a given node. These retrieval requests were introduced already in chapter 5. In the following, more details about their circuitires will be discussed, and the ways that they are combined into more elaborated retrieval requests will be outlined

A **hint** is a retrieval request that specifies a set of nodes to be retrieved by their **semantic relationship** with a given set of nodes, which are called the **root of the hint**. In this context, semantic relationship would mean any relationship except AND and OR. Quite often, the root of a hint consists of only one node. Hints can be combined to more complex retrieval request by **set-operators** such as intersection ($\bigcap$) and union ($\bigcup$). The set-operators operate on the sets of nodes that are defined by the hints. Consider, for example, the retrieval request: "find an exemplar of the classes 'transportation-means' and 'is-on-the-water'". 'Exemplar of the class transportation means' is a hint. Its root is the class 'transportation means', which defines the set whose members are car, airplane, boat, etc. The semantic relationship in this hint is 'exemplar of the class'. 'Is on the water' is the second hint. Its root is 'the water', and its semantic relationship is 'is-on'. In this example, the two hints are combined by 'and', which, when dealing with the set-operators, is 'intersection'.

After introducing notations that can be used to express retrieval requests, some basic circuitries that can perform retrievals will be described.

Notations

Let $\{G\}=\{g_1,...,g_n\}$ denote a set of nodes G whose members are nodes g_i, $i=1,...,n$, where n is the number of nodes in the set. Let REL denote a semantic relational concept, which defines a relationship between concept nodes.

The expression $\{REL(g_i)\}$ defines the set of nodes that have the relationship REL with g_i. For example, $\{is\text{-}part\text{-}of(g_i)\}$ is the set of nodes that are parts of g_i.

Since expressions of the form $\{REL(g_i)\}$ define sets, they can be used in conjunction with set-operators. For example, the expression $\{R\} = \bigcap_{i=1}^{n}\{is\text{-}item\text{-}of(g_i)\}$ defines a set $\{R\}$, whose members are nodes, which may be denoted by r_j. Each r_j is an item-node to which the g_i's (all n of them) belong as parts.

The expression $\{REL\{G\}\}$ defines a set whose members are obtained by REL operating on each member of $\{G\}$: $\{REL\{G\}\} \equiv \bigcup_{i=1}^{n}\{REL(g_i)\}$.

A chain of relational concepts can operate on a node or on a set of nodes: $\{REL_1 \cdot REL_2\{G\}\} \equiv \{REL_1\{REL_2\{G\}\}\}$.

Expressions of the type: $\{REL(g_i)\}$, $\{REL\{G\}\}$, and $\{REL_1 \cdots REL_m\{G\}\}$ are **hints**. For example, the hint $\{is\text{-}class\text{-}of(g_i)\}$

defines the set whose members are class-nodes that have g_1 as their exemplar. The hint {is-exemplar-of{is-class-of(g_1)}} defines a set of exemplar-nodes that belong to the classes of which g_1 is an exemplar too.

A fundamental hint consists of a fundamental relationship that operates on one node. The fundamental relationships are is-a-class-of, is-an-exemplar-of, is-an-item-of, and is-a-part-of. Fundamental-hint and fundamental-request are synonyms.

In the following, the set-operator 'not', will be considered a semantic relationship, which is a part of a hint.

When a retrieval request operates on an actual memory, which consists of inter-related nodes, it may retrieve one node (a singleton set), a set of several nodes, or no node at all (the empty set), depending on the memory's contents.

Retrieval requests are basic building blocks of thinking processes. A thinking unit has means to compile such retrieval requests and to execute them. A variety of hardware implementation can be devised for handling retrieval requests. Several types of such circuitries are described next.

Fundamental retrievers

A fundamental retriever is a circuitry that retrieves a target that is specified by a fundamental hint (a hint consisting of one given node (g), whose specified relationship with the target is one of the four fundamental relationships: g is-a-class-of?, g is-an-exemplar-of?, g is-an-item-of?, or g is-a-part-of?). Limits on the expected number of retrieved nodes may be specified in the retrieval request. The inter-relationships between the major sub-units of a possible fundamental retriever are illustrated in figure 7.1. This fundamental retriever employs the following strategy: First, the node g is latched onto the given-slot sub-unit. This can be accomplished by establishing a temporary exemplar-class connection between the two. The control bundles of g are latched to the iterator sub-unit. The modulation factors of the bundles of g are then set according to the retrieval request. (The data bundle that corresponds to the specified relationship is enabled, while the other data bundles are disabled.) The activation factor of the enabled bundle is initially set to very close to zero. The requesting routine then activates the trigger, which activates the iterator and concurrently causes the firing of node g and the labeling of its output. At first, nodes S1 and S2 may not be activated. The iterator increases the modulation factor, and at the same time keeps superimposing a label on the outgoing signals. Eventually, nodes S1 and S2 will fire and will be labeled. They will be

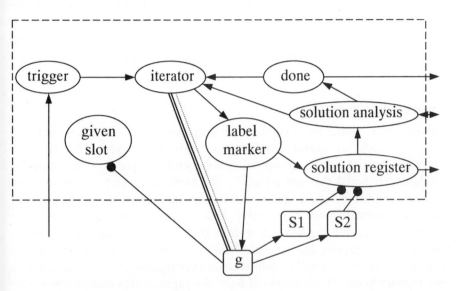

Figure 7.1: The sub-units of a fundamental retriever (inside the dashed frame). Arrows indicate direction of information flow. The trigger of the routine activates the iterator. Bundles from the iterator control and detect the activities of the modulators and of the core of the given node (g). They also activate the label marker, which sends labels to bundles of the given node and to the solution register. The labels pass on to the retrieved nodes (nodes S1 and S2), and facilitate the establishment of connections between them and the solution register. The solution analysis sub-unit decides whether to continue the iteration or to stop it, in which case it signals the done sub-unit.

recognized by the solution-detector sub-unit, which has received the key to the label from the label marker. If the number of solutions is acceptable (could be determined from the total intensity of the detected activity), a signal is sent from the solution-detector to the done sub-unit. If the detected activity is below or above expectations, appropriate signals are sent from the solution-detector to the iterator sub-unit. The iterator adjusts the modulation factor as needed, and continues looping. Such iterations are terminated by a signal from the 'done' sub-unit, or by an external signal, e.g. in cases when the iterations have been going on for too long. This retrieval strategy will first retrieve nodes with the largest weights from node g. As the iteration progresses, nodes with lesser weights will be retrieved too. Only nodes that are directly connected with node g can be retrieved. Because of the transitivity of the four fundamental relationships, nodes that satisfy the retrieval request may be connected to g indirectly. Such nodes can be retrieved by a chain of simple retrieval requests, e.g. {the-class-of{the-class-of(g)}}.

Serial fundamental retrievers

Fundamental retrievers become sub-units of more complex retrieval requests, such as **serial fundamental retrievers**. Serial fundamental requests consist of a group of fundamental requests (the same as fundamental hints) that are joined by the same set operator. The retrieval strategy employed by the serial fundamental retriever is to execute each of the fundamental hints separately, and to accumulate their union or intersection set in a register. (A register is a class node that is permanently connected to circuits that execute basic operations of the system. To be placed in a register, a node establishes an exemplar-to-class connection with the register node. To be removed from the register, this connection is cut-off.) At the end of the process, any node left at the register will be a solution to the retrieval request. If the memory does not contain any solution, the register will be empty. The unit that executes this strategy will be called a **serial fundamental retriever**.

Figure 7.2 outlines the sub-units of a serial fundamental retriever, and the role of its fundamental-retriever sub-unit. It illustrates how a node or nodes are retrieved that satisfy a retrieval request of the form $\{R\} = \bigcap_{i,j}\{REL_j(g_{ij})\}$, where the REL_j are fundamental relations. Each retrieved node, which belongs to {R}, satisfies all the fundamental requests of the right hand side.

Fundamental hints are first processed by a fundamental retriever. Then, the set-operation sub-unit operates on the retrieved hints. The first retrieved hint is transferred to the accumulator. Then, the next retrieved hint is loaded into the hints register. Its intersection with the set that is already stored in accumulator is found, and remains in the accumulator. (Only nodes that are exemplars of both the accumulator and the hints register remain in the accumulator). This strategy ensures that only correct solutions remain in the accumulator when the entire retrieval request is completed.

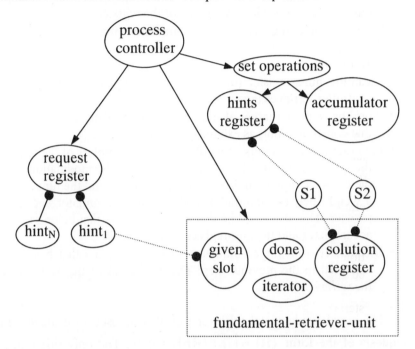

Figure 7.2: A serial fundamental retriever. Initially, the fundamental hint requests are stored at the request register. The process controller causes a hint to be loaded to the given slot of the fundamental-retriever-unit, and it then activates that unit. That unit retrieves its target and places it at the solution register. Once the done sub-unit fires, indicating that the target of the hint was retrieved, the process controller causes the solution nodes to be loaded from the solution slot of the fundamental retriever to the hints register. The set operation sub-unit then causes the appropriate transfer of information from the hint register to the accumulator. The same process is executed on the next hint in the request register, until all the hints are processed.

The steps of the execution of the request $\{hint_1\} \bigcap \{hint_2\}$ are as follows (also illustrated in figure 7.3):

- Clear the hints-register and the accumulator (disconnect all the exemplars).

- Copy the retrieved target from the solution slot of the fundamental-retriever-unit to the hints-register. (Make the nodes that constitute the retrieved target of $hint_1$ exemplars of the register).
- Copy the hints-register to the accumulator (make the nodes that are exemplars of the hint-register become also exemplars of the accumulator).
- Clear the hints-register (disconnect its exemplars). Now, the process-controller retrieves the target of $hint_2$.
- Store the retrieved target of $hint_2$ in the hint-register (connect the nodes that constitute $hint_2$ as exemplars of the register).
- Find (activate) the intersection of the set of exemplars of the register and the set of exemplars of the accumulator. (Set the modulation factors in the class-exemplar bundles of the accumulator and the hints-register to a weight between 0.5 and 1, and fire the accumulator and the hints-register. The result will be that only exemplars that belong to both the accumulator and the hint-register will fire.)
- Disconnect from the accumulator all the exemplars that have not been activated in the previous step. The exemplars of the accumulator are the retrieved nodes.

The serial fundamental retriever can also be used to evaluate retrieval requests of the form $\{R\} = \bigcup_{i,j}\{REL_j(g_{ij})\}$. The only difference from the previous retrieval request would be that now the set-operations sub-unit would perform a union operation as it incorporates the nodes in the hints register and the accumulator. In figure 7.3, frame 5, the accumulator will inhibit all its nodes, while the hints register will send activating signals to all its nodes. Only non-inhibited nodes will fire, and will be added to the accumulator.

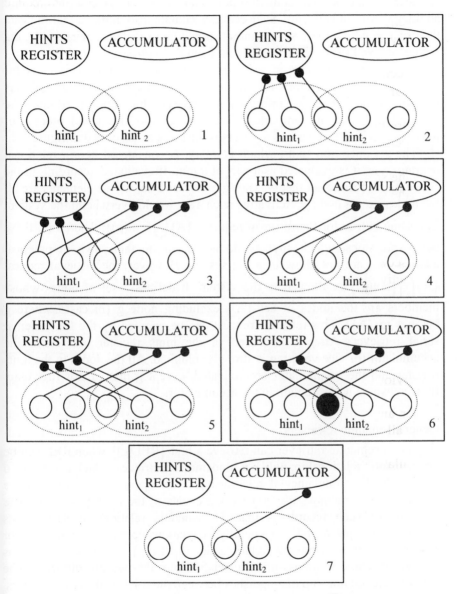

Figure 7.3: Executing the retrieval request $\{hint_1\} \bigcap \{hint_2\}$ – the
interactions between the hints register and the accumulator.

Retrievers containing combinations of AND, OR, and NOT

Retrieval requests that contain both 'and' and 'or' operations require additional control elements. Such requests contain also markers that indicate the order in which these set-operators should be executed. For example, the request <A.and.<B.or.C>> is different from the request <<A.and.B>.or.C> , where the arrow brackets < > indicate order of operation. This calls for temporary storage locations for intermediary results. A specialized unit has to direct the flow of information between the hint registers, the accumulators, and the temporary storage locations. The actual process of moving data between various registers is the same as described in figure 7.3.

The set operation 'not', which is unary, is considered here a relational operator, and it is evaluated as a part of a hint. If evaluated according to the convention of finite-set theory, $\{not(g)\}$ defines a set whose elements are all the nodes except node g. Activating such a set would overwhelm the system. The same is true for the retrieval request $\{A\}\bigcup\{not(g)\}$. Therefore, these two expressions, which anyhow do not occur on their own in practical applications, are not allowed in the system. However, the retrieval request $\{A\}\bigcap\{not(g)\}$ is allowed in the system. It defines a set of nodes whose members are the nodes of set $\{A\}$, excluding node g (in cases where g belongs to $\{A\}$). This retrieval request can be handled by the fundamental serial retriever. After g is stored in the hints register and A in the accumulator (or vice versa), g is strongly inhibited. All the nodes in the hints register and the accumulator are activated, except g that cannot fire. Only these activated nodes remain in the accumulator.

General semantic retrievers

A general semantic retriever can retrieve a hint $\{REL(g)\}$ when REL can be any semantic relationship, unlike a fundamental retriever, which is limited to one of the four fundamental relationships. Its operation is based on the format that the memory uses for storing events of the form (h,REL,g). The meaning of such records is that the semantic relationship REL exists between concepts h and g. Generally, a relationship can be symmetric or asymmetric. In a symmetric relationship, (h,REL,g) is the same event as (g,REL,h), while in an asymmetric relationship, the two are different. The asymmetric relationship distinguishes between the roles of the two variables. The following is a circuitry of a general semantic retriever for both symmetric and asymmetric relationships.

The way that experienced relationships are stored in the memory facilitates the retrieval of the set {REL(g)}, when the root-node g and the relational concept REL are specified. Assume that a certain relational concept REL was found to exist between pairs of concept nodes (g_i,h_i) i=1,...m. The memory records encode the fact that each of these pairs happened as a part of a corresponding event (h_i,REL,g_i). At the center of each record is a class node, designated as REL in figure 7.4. The exemplars of REL are nodes that represent the m pairs. Each node that represents a pair has the corresponding elements g_i and h_i as its parts. If REL is asymmetric, all the g_i's are exemplars of a class node 'the first variable of REL' (VAR1), and all the h_i's are exemplars of the class node VAR2. Figure 7.4 illustrates the situation for m=2.

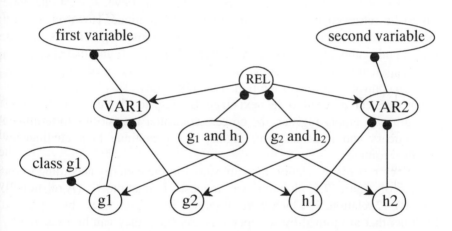

Figure 7.4: Circuitry of the memory records (h_1RELg_1) and (h_2RELg_2). Usually, nodes g_1, g_2, h_1, and h_2 are instances of their corresponding classes. Only the class-node that represents class g_1 is shown.

The following operations take place in retrieving {REL(g_1)}. They are performed by a dedicated circuitry, which consists of fundamental-retrieval circuitries. They operate on data structures that are stored as shown in figure 7.4. The general retrieval strategy consists of a chain of fundamental retrievers that were described above. The output of one retriever serves as input to the next (piped operations). The operations are: First, retrieve VAR1. Second, retrieve all the nodes that represent pairs (g_1 and h_i). Third, retrieve all the h_i's. The individual operations are:

- VAR1={an-exemplar-of(first-variable)} $\bigcap$ {a-part-of(REL)}.   This retrieves VAR1.

- g_i={an-exemplar-of(VAR1)} $\bigcap$ {an-exemplar-of(class g_i)}.   Retrieves all the instances of g_i that were first variables of REL.

- {g_i and h_i}= {an-item-of(g_i)} $\bigcap$ {an-exemplar-of(REL)}.   Retrieves all the nodes that represent pairs that have g_i as their first variable.

- {h_i}= {a-part-of{g_i and h_i}} $\bigcap$ {not(g_i)} Retrieves all the h_i's.

If the relationship REL is symmetric, there are no VAR1 and VAR2 nodes in the representations of the events.

In various stages of all the processes described above, at least one node has to be retrieved in order for the process to continue. However, certain memories may not contain any node that satisfies those requirements, and so, such a node cannot be retrieved. A **register-flag** is a sub-unit that checks if a register is empty or it has some information. It is activated as part of the process control, and fires if the register is not empty. This firing signals that the process can proceed to the next stage. If a register-flag does not fire, thus indicating an empty register, the process controller may decide to terminate the process and issue an error signal, or to continue in a contingency retrieval routine.

When records of relationships are stored in the memory according to the format of figure 7.4, the retrieval requests (?,relation,B), (A,relation,?), (A,?,B), (?,relation,?), which were discussed in chapter 4, can be expressed by hints that are joined by set operators. As such, they can be executed by the circuitries described above. The request (?A,relation,B?), which means: "is there a record of (A,relation,B) in the memory?" can be expressed as {A,relation,?} $\bigcap$ (B). Firing of the register-flag of the accumulator at the end of the process encodes the answer 'yes'.

Scanners

Scanning is a common process in the thinking system. When a node is scanned, nodes that are related to it in a certain way are retrieved one at a time. The scanning process, which involves several sub-units, is controlled by a scanning-controller node. The currently retrieved node is made available to the scanning-controller, which decides whether to continue the scanning or to terminate it. Scanning ends when there are no more nodes to retrieve, or when a retrieved node meets the scanning goal. Figure 7.5 illustrates the sub-units of a possible scanner.

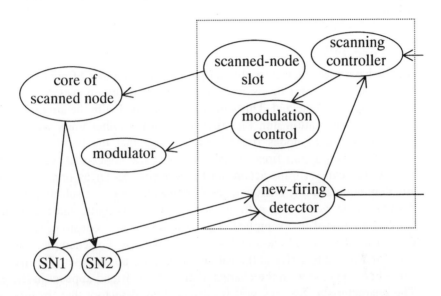

Figure 7.5: Sub-units that participate in scanning the parts of the scanned node.

The sub-units of a scanner are shown inside the dashed box in figure 7.5. The outcomes of scanning the core of the given node are nodes SN1 and then SN2. SN1 is the first node to be retrieved, and SN2 is the second. The scanner disables all the modulators of the bundles of the scanned node, except one (item-to-parts in this case) that is set to a very small value. The scanner latches to the core of the scanned node, and keeps it firing throughout the entire process. It instructs the modulation control unit to gradually increase the modulation factor. Eventually, SN1 will fire. Two main factors determine which node will fire first. The first factor is the synaptic weight between the scanned node and its part-nodes. The second factor is prior priming of the part-nodes. Part-nodes may get input from other nodes, in additional to what they get from the scanned node. When the overall core potential, which is the sum of the modulated signals from the scanned node and from those other nodes, passes the threshold, the part-node will fire. That will be detected by the new-firing-detector, which will mark

SN1 as the newly retrieved node, and notify the controller. If the controller decides to continue the scanning, it instructs the modulation-control sub-unit to continue. Node SN2 will eventually fire, be marked for the initiator, and so on.

Traps and anticipation

Arenas have many detectors that monitor a large number of nodes. In some situations, the system needs to be notified when certain patterns of firing nodes have been detected. This can be accomplished with the aid of a trap. A **trap** is a computation unit that fires and notifies other units when a pre-selected pattern of nodes fires (it can be said that the firing pattern was trapped). When a trap fires, it also identifies the nodes that were trapped. The system can set traps according to its needs. As far as implementation, any item node and any class node can serve as the detector sub-unit of a trap. An item node would trap patterns that consist of its parts, and a class node would trap any of its exemplars. The system may also construct specialized circuitries of item and class nodes to serve as traps. For example, when we wait for a friend to arrive at the gate in the airport, a trap is set. This trap will fire when a person with the characteristics of our friend appears in the gate. The characteristic features will be detected by detectors that, in turn, will activate the trap. The firing trap will direct our attention to the cause of its firing–the image of our friend. Traps can also be set for concepts that are stored in the memory. When the memory is scanned, the trap fires as a desired concept is activated. This may serve as an indication to a scanning controller to finish the scanning.

Some traps operate in passive mode. They won't send out any signals until they have detected the presence of their target. Other traps would send out signals, indicating that they are set and that they are expecting certain things to happen. If those signals are sent to awareness detectors, the system becomes aware of the trap. This is how the model represents the feeling of anticipation. If the trap sends signals also to feeling nodes, such as nodes that represent joy, fear, uncertainty, and so on, the anticipation is perceived as pleasant or unpleasant. The intensity of those feelings may build up with time, and may eventually cause the dismantling of the trap. Sometimes, upon detecting the presence of its target, the signal that is sent out by the trap invokes a positive feeling of relief or satisfaction.

Action-outcome routines

The scope of action-outcome routines

The goal of action-outcome routines is to preserve the well being of the system. They are triggered when certain key concepts are detected in incoming stimuli. If a threat to the system is detected, an action-outcome routine on ways to eliminate or to avoid it would be triggered. If a beneficial situation is detected, the triggered action-outcome routine would guide the system in preserving or enhancing the situation. Action-outcome routines are usually under the control of authorization programs, which enable the execution of the actions prescribed by the action-outcome routines. If the execution is not enabled, the triggered action-outcome routine remains a thought.

One of the simplest action-outcome routines is the reflex. Generally, a reflex is an activation flow that associates a cue with an action. Once a cue is detected in the incoming data, an action of the system is invoked. The system expects that the invoked action would be followed by a desired outcome, which is not under direct control of the system. In simple reflexes, a given cue will always invoke the same action. In elaborate reflexes, the system considers, in addition to the cue, other variables that specify the state of the system and the environment. For example, when inadvertently we touch a hot object, a reflex will withdraw our hand back. The sensation of heat is the cue that triggers the reflex. However, the actual withdrawal is based on additional information. If the hand approached the hot object from above, it will be withdrawn upward. If it approached the object from below, the withdrawal will be downwards. Other than the cue, the system has also considered the history of the event. This information may have been encoded as certain motor neurons being active. The reflex caused the activation of neurons that control antagonistic movements. In all these cases, the action was expected to follow by a desired outcome, which is the cessation of the pain.

With time, the system adds to its innate reflexes new action-outcome routines, so that it could better preserve its well being when new situations arise. These action-outcome routines may be encoded directly by dedicated circuitries, which invoke the appropriate action in a reflexive manner. However, the system may also use general procedures that provide a temporary action-outcome circuitry when needs arise, based on memory records of previous experiences. Temporary routines become permanent if their circuitry is preserved. Usually, both kinds of action-outcome routines are capable of handling situations that differ from the actual experiences on which they are based.

Action-outcome routines operate in steps. The coordination between the steps may be autonomous or it may be done by external controllers. Executed steps in an autonomous routine trigger the execution of subsequent steps. Controllers, on the other hand, are units that can coordinate the activities of various unrelated routines. The controllers base their instructions on general information that they receive from the executing routines.

Action-outcome routines have three components: actions, outcomes, and flags. Actions are those activities that are initiated by the routine. They include activating motor units and projectors, activating retrieval requests, and setting traps. The second component–the outcomes–consists of internal and external consequences of the actions. They are detected by the circuitry of the action-outcome routine. They include data retrieved from the memory, data extracted from the flow initiated by external stimuli, and data extracted by detectors from projected scenes. The third component–flags–are indications about the status of the ongoing activities of the step. They include indications that the expected outcome is available, not available, or cannot be obtained. They also include an indication that the end of the action-outcome routine was reached. The flags that are activated during the execution of a step and the resulting outcomes determine the next step that will be executed by the routine. The outcomes obtained in one step may serve as input to the following steps. The last step of an action-outcome routine is the reaction to the original trigger. Steps may be nested within each other. A nested step is a sub-routine of its nesting step. The outcome of the sub-routine is an intermediate goal on the way to the goal of the nesting step.

The system uses general procedures to generate an action-outcome circuitry based upon memory records of relevant experiences. Consider the following situation as an example. In hot summer days, cows in a pasture seem to know to move to the shade. The following is a hypothetical record of events, as recorded in a cow's brain: a sensation of feeling too hot, the head looks around, the big oak tree is spotted, the gaze is locked on the big oak tree, the body moves toward the tree, the body enters the shade, and the sensation of relief from the heat. Figure 7.6 describes a portion of the memory record of the event, based on which the first step of an action-outcome routine could be generated. It records the sensation of feeling too hot, looking around, and seeing the big oak tree.

An action-outcome circuitry based on this memory record needs several additional sub-units. It needs a trigger that activates the circuitry when the external conditions call for it. It needs a sub-unit that activates the motor units, which execute the looking around, and it needs a sub-unit that evaluates the signals from the visual scenery. The latter indicates when the step has achieved its goal, and the next step in the sequence (moving towards the shade) should begin.

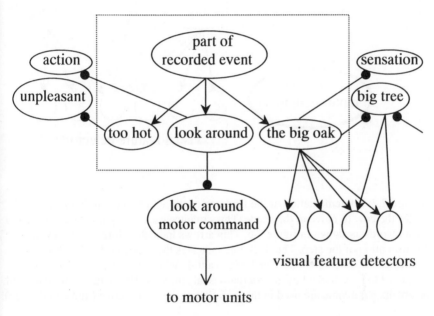

Figure 7.6: The memory record of the event (inside the dashed line): 'It was too hot. While looking around, the big oak tree was seen', and how it relates to some other memory nodes, and to the node that activates the motor units of looking around.

Figure 7.7 illustrates an action-outcome circuitry, which is based on the data record of figure 7.6. This circuitry executes the step of looking around when it is too hot, until the big oak is seen. The trigger of the action-outcome routine is 'sensation of too hot'. The action is 'look around', and the outcome is 'see the big oak tree'. This circuitry can be generated from the data record (figure 7.6) by a general-purpose construction routine, whose elements are retrieval requests of the kinds that were described at the beginning of this chapter. Following is the description of that construction routine, and how it is implemented in this particular case.

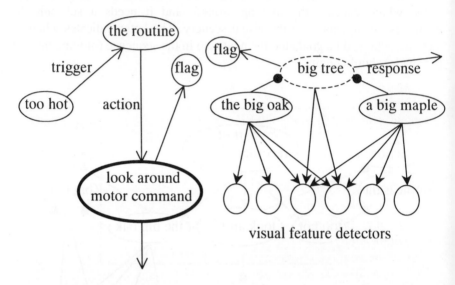

Figure 7.7: Implementation of the first step of the action-outcome routine, which guides the cow to move to the shade. This circuitry uses as a template the format of data records as shown in figure 7.6. Thin arrows indicate information flow during the execution of the step. The thick line indicates the action node. The dashed line indicates the outcome node. The latter is a trap, which is set by the routine and is supposed to be activated by an external visual stimulus. The status of the flags and the obtained outcome are used in the initiation of the next routine (move to the tree).

Constructing action-outcome routines

The need for an action-outcome routine is initiated by a state of the system. If the state is unpleasant, the routine should get the system out of it, and if the state is pleasant, the routine should preserve the situation. Consider, without loss of generality, an unpleasant situation. The construction routine goes through the following steps:

- Find a node (A) which is an exemplar of unpleasant feeling and which is present now (i.e. exemplar of the class 'currently active node'). In the example above, the retrieved node A would be 'too hot'.
- Find a node (B) which contains A as a part, and which contains 'A is eliminated' as another part. In the example above B would be the memory record of the event: "a sensation of feeling too hot, the head looks around, the big oak tree is spotted, the gaze is locked on the big oak tree, the body moves toward the tree, the body enters the shade, and the **sensation of relief from the heat**".
- Find a node (C), which is a part of 'B', and which contains the following nodes as its parts: 'A'; an exemplar of 'action' (D); and an exemplar of 'sensation' (E). In the example above, C would be 'part of recorded event' (figure 7.6), D would be 'look around', and E would be 'the big oak'.
- Find an activator of motor units (F), whose exemplar is D. In the example above that would be 'look around motor command'.
- Find a class node (G), whose exemplar is E. In the example above that would be 'big tree. In this step, 'big tree' is set as a trap. It would respond to 'the big oak', and to other big trees. That would be a generalization of the original situation, which is a desired quality of an action-outcome routine.
- Recruit nodes to represent the program and the flags (figure 7.7), and connect them to the nodes that have been retrieved in the previous steps. That terminates the construction of the first step of the action-outcome routine.

This set of procedures is quite general, and it can be used to construct steps in a variety of situations that require an action-outcome routine. These procedures rely only on the retrieval requests processes that were described earlier.

In general, replacing the node that represents the actual outcome by its class-node (as was done in the fifth step above) provides the action-outcome routine with a broader trap. The routine will respond not only to a recurrence of the original outcome, but also to other outcomes, which are exemplars of the same class. The same thing is true for replacing the actual action by its class node, when selecting the action node of a step. This kind of generalization can be applied to the elements of any step in an action-outcome routine. Since a node may be an exemplar of many classes, such generalizations of a given memory record are not unique. Different action-outcome routines may be constructed from a given memory record. A higher level program supervises the construction of such routines. It evaluates the performance of a routine and decides if there is a need to construct another one.

An action-outcome routine may be recorded directly, as an autonomous action-outcome routine, even without keeping a distinct record of the experienced event itself. In other words, the system may have a circuitry like figure 7.7, without having a circuitry like figure 7.6. In such cases, the cow would go reflexively to a tree, without being able to recall the experience on which this action is based.

Usually, when confronted with a situation, the system will first attempt to use an existing action-outcome routine. If none exists, or if the outcome of an employed routine has been unsatisfactory, the system would try to construct a temporary routine from relevant memory records. Any memory record that contains the same trigger as the current situation combined with a satisfactory response to it can serve as a potential template for the action-outcome routine. Temporary action-outcome routines may become permanent if they have produced good results.

Action-outcome routines and the system

Action-outcome routines are being extended and updated all the time. Crying is a very early action-outcome routine, which is employed by a newborn for getting food and drink. With time, a baby's memory will have records of various situations that can serve as templates for achieving the goal of thirst quenching. Children further increase their repertoire and acquire routines that guide them in situations that are more complex. For example, they learn to respect drinks that belong to others, to buy drinks, and so on. Not all of these are stand-alone routines. Action-outcome routines act concurrently and interdependently with other routines. Respecting property of others is a basic routine that is always on, at least to some extent. It will indicate that taking somebody else's drink may cause problems. This information, together with the information from an action-outcome routine for drinking, is provided to a higher-level routine, which coordinates the activities of the system.

Many action-outcome routines, which are supposed to prompt responses in unfamiliar situations, are based on limited experiences of the system. Consequently, a novel situation may trigger several action-outcome routines that may prompt conflicting actions. For example, the smell of a piece of cheese would prompt a mouse's system to approach it. The sight of a cat would prompt the mouse to freeze or to flee. Eventually, a mouse may find itself in a scene that contains both a cat and a piece of cheese. The two action-outcome routines will be activated concurrently, and will point to conflicting actions. Systems may use different mechanisms to reach a decision in such circumstances. The simplest would be if each possible response had a weight, and in cases of conflict, the strongest prevails. Hardware implementations of this mechanism are relatively simple. One possibility is to have a decision center that is activated when conflicts arise. It neutralizes the weak response, and leaves only the strongest. A more complex mechanism would expand the search for additional responses when conflicts occur. It would look for a response that creates the most pleasant outcomes, and avoids the unpleasant ones. That may require an extensive scanning of exemplars and substituting them in the exemplar slots of the proposed action-outcome routines. The scanning will stop when the substituted exemplars will not prompt conflicting actions.

Drives

Types of drives

In psychology, drives are defined as the internal forces behind actions or desires. Primary drives exist in the system from birth or become part of it in predetermined growth processes. Secondary drives are developed based on individual experiences. Different psychological theories suggest different hierarchies of primary and secondary drives as explanations for observed behavior patterns. The model does not endorse or reject any of these theories. Rather, it provides generic circuitries that can support any hierarchy of primary and secondary drives. In the model, drives can be represented by standard circuitry–usually as action-outcome routines.

When a drive is represented by an action-outcome routine, the last expected outcome of the routine represents the goal of the drive. One way of classifying drives is by the type of their goals. Homeostatic drives are primary drives that maintain the internal environment of the body at an appropriate constant state. They include feeding and drinking drives, temperature regulation drives, and the likes. These drives are triggered by well-defined unpleasant stimuli, and the goal of the drives is to eliminate the unpleasant triggering effects. Other primary drives, such as sexual and parenting drives, are triggered by stimuli that are not necessarily unpleasant. The outcomes of these drives cover the entire gamut of pleasant-unpleasant feelings. In some cases, a pleasant outcome is hardwired into the system, so that the organism is automatically rewarded after the completion of the drive. In some cases, an external source provides a pleasant reward. In other cases, no specific feeling is expected to follow the completion of the drive.

Primary drives may be expanded by all kinds of experiences, while retaining their original nature. For example, a man's or a woman's primary sexual drive consists of a sequence of steps, each having its trigger, its action, and its expected outcome. An outcome of one step serves as the trigger of the next. Although the main physiological components of the sexual act are almost identical among all men and among all women, there is great individual variability in the triggers, in the details of the actions, and in the expected outcomes. It is suggested that individual experiences induce the creation of new circuitries that are added to the original ones. Many of the experiences that expand the triggers and the expected outcomes occur before the sexual maturity of the individual. Although they are not experiences of direct sexual activity, they affect the expansion of the original sex drive. Expansions of the action parts of the sex drive are based mainly on sexual experiences, which are gained after puberty.

The system may find out that certain intermediate outcomes, which are reached in the execution of a primary drive, would eventually lead to the original goal of that drive. These outcomes then become precursors of rewards. As such, they may become goals of new secondary drives, which the system adopts. These secondary drives may develop triggers of their own, which are different from the triggers of the original drives. For example, sooner or later we realize that having money makes it easier to satisfy the needs behind many of our drives, such as food, thirst, comfortable temperature, and so on. Having money then becomes a recognized reward and a goal of a secondary drive. This secondary drive has its own trigger, which is usually not the sensation of hunger, thirst, or cold. In general, experiences that lead to gratification or to avoidance of displeasure may be transformed into drives on their own. The needs to be gratified and to avoid displeasure seem to be primary drives that can be expanded easily.

Circuitry of drives

A one-step primary drive consists of several sub-units: a trigger, an action sub-unit, which executes the drive, and a controller, which coordinates between the status of the trigger, the activities, and the outcome. A multi-step drive consists of a sequence of steps, each having an action and an outcome sub-unit. An intermediate step may be triggered solely by a signal indicating that the preceding step has been completed, or by a combination of such a signal and an external trigger. The controller of a multi-step drive has circuitry that orchestrates the execution of the steps. It activates the activation sub-units and sets the traps of the outcome sub-units in the right sequence and according to the outside triggers. It also prevents completed steps from repeating themselves, even if their triggers are still present. A drive would terminate its own action if the sub-unit that detects the last outcome–the goal–sends a signal to the drive-controller that it has been achieved. Figure 7.8 illustrates the main sub-units of a multi-step drive circuitry.

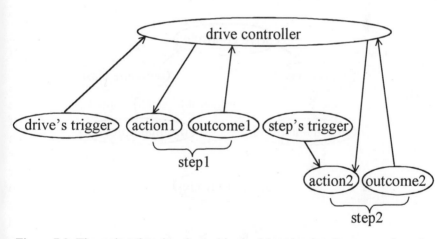

Figure 7.8: The main sub-units of a multi-step drive circuitry (two steps shown). Arrows indicate direction of information flow.

A drive's circuitry can be expanded in many ways. It would retain its original nature if its first trigger and its expected last outcome remain unchanged, while all the changes affect intermediate sub-units. For example, the feeding drive of an animal would retain its original nature as long as it and its expansion are triggered by the sensation of hunger, and are terminated by the outcome sensation of being sate. The original feeding drive may have an intermediate step in which the action is to move and to sniff, and the related expected outcome is a certain odor. That action sub-unit may be expanded to include looking around and scanning the area, and its outcome sub-unit may be expanded to include also the sight of certain fruits. These changes will not change the nature of the drive. Nodes that represent the expanded action and the expanded outcome are added to the original nodes.

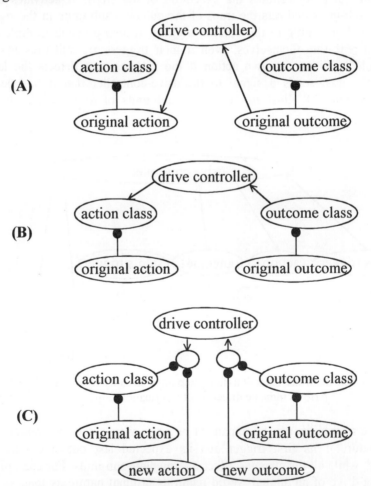

Figure 7.9: An original step of a drive (part A), and two of its expansions.

Figure 7.9 illustrates two general ways in which a step of an original drive (A) can be expanded. First (B), the controller swaps its connection to the original action node with the class node of the original action, and/or swaps its connection to the original outcome with the class node of that original outcome. That would make the step more general. For example, if the taste of honey were the original outcome in a certain feeding drive, replacing the 'honey' node by its class-node 'sweet' would expand the drive without changing its nature. All the co-exemplars of that class node, including the original outcome, would be treated by the drive's circuitry as expected outcomes. Similarly, action nodes could also be expanded by swapping an action node by one of its class nodes.

If a trigger of a drive and/or its last outcome are expanded, the nature of the drive changes. It gets a different cause and/or a different goal. In such cases, a primary drive develops a secondary offshoot, and a secondary drive develops an additional secondary offshoot. Hardware mechanisms that bring about these changes are shown in part (C) of figure 7.9. A drive may develop a different goal when an intermediary outcome, which is not part of the original circuitry, is frequently associated with the original goal. This intermediary outcome then becomes the goal of a secondary offshoot drive. As mentioned earlier, after noticing that 'money' is associated with the original goal 'becoming sate', 'money' becomes the goal of a secondary drive to get money. Just being awake may be the trigger to this new drive. With time, the new drive to get money expands, as the individual adopts new actions and expected outcomes, which should lead to achieving the new goal.

Learning of drives

By their nature, drives are intended to be expanded. They have to operate in changing environments, whose exact details could not be foreseen at the outset of the system. The system has mechanisms that control how existing drives are affected by experiences, and how new drives are acquired. The mechanisms of expanding drives are based on addition of new nodes as exemplars or classes to existing circuitry–operations that are supported by the model. **Learning-control-sub-units** (LCSUs) coordinate the use of these basic operations in the expansion and the modification of existing drives. An LCSU is triggered when an experience that warrants learning occurs. For example, the termination of an unpleasant feeling, which a drive is supposed to regulate, can trigger the LCSU of that drive. The LCSU would have to identify the cause of the change and update the drive's circuitry accordingly. The cause may be an action of the system or some external factor. A new action should update an action node of the drive, and an external factor should update an outcome node of the drive (figure 7.9). The LCSU marks the involved nodes and coordinates the formation of new appropriate connections between them. Usually, the LCSU would not have precise information about the true cause of the termination of the unpleasant feeling, because the true cause may be hidden in irrelevant stimuli. In order to separate the true cause and utilize it, the LCSU would have to rely on compare-and-contrast learning mechanisms, which are supported by the system (chapter 5).

The termination of unpleasant feelings or the enhancements of pleasant ones are not always the only trigger of the LCSU of the corresponding drive. For example, during the pre-puberty period, some learning and expansions of the sexual drive are not triggered by sexually pleasant or unpleasant experiences. A large variety of experiences, which involve external sensations and internal feelings, appear to be able to trigger the LCSU of the sexual drive. One possibility is that the innate LCSU of the sex drive is already wired to be triggered by that variety of stimuli. Another possibility is that the trigger is innately wired to be triggered only by sexual experiences, but it becomes expanded by other experiences, and eventually other stimuli can trigger it. It is not exactly clear which experiences trigger this LCSU, and what mechanisms it uses to separate the 'relevant' from the 'irrelevant' information and to record it.

The process of developing secondary drives, which have new goals, may be divided into two. First, a new goal (e.g. getting money, pleasing a parent) becomes an exemplar of the class of rewarding outcomes. This can be accomplished through the process of conditioning (chapter 5). Then, action-outcome routines to accomplish that goal are established based on experiences, as described in the previous section.

Curiosity and novelty

It is believed that curiosity is one of the basic drives of humans and other animals. Quite often, the sensation of a new or unfamiliar situation is the trigger of curiosity. However, it is possible that curiosity is a basic drive that does not need an external trigger, and one of its reward is the sensation of 'new'. Both propositions could be handled by the model. 'New' is one of the fundamental concepts of the model. Novelty detection is based on comparing incoming stimuli with records of past experiences. It is rare that an incoming pattern would match exactly a recorded one. Usually, an incoming pattern would have new sub-patterns and familiar ones.

A sub-pattern may be declared 'new' due to nodes and/or connections that it has that are not contained in any recorded pattern. However, novelty detectors may classify as 'familiar' patterns that contain new sub-patterns. The key to novelty classification is comparing the entire data structure of the incoming pattern with recorded data structures. An incoming pattern is parsed by various detectors, and its features are organized as a data structure consisting of basic concepts and basic relationships. If significant parts of the data structure of the incoming pattern have been matched with a recorded data structure, the incoming pattern is considered familiar. If, on the other hand, some critical elements of the information structures did not find a match or were involved in a conflict, the incoming stimulus is classified as 'new', and the curiosity drive may be triggered.

When triggered by a novelty detector, the action component of the curiosity drive initiates activities that should provide more information about the new stimulus. These include motor activities that manipulate the relationships between the stimulus and the system (e.g. moving around a new object to get more information about it), and mental activities that search the memory for records associated with the stimulus. Usually, these mental activities are standard thinking operations. The expected outcome of those activities is that the new stimulus becomes familiar. When that happens, curiosity fades. A stimulus becomes familiar when it is incorporated into the database of the system. It may get a new item node, and, through the activities of the detectors of the system, it develops standard ties with other existing nodes.

Brain Operation Supervisor (BOS)

Responsibilities of a BOS

Drives, impulses, action-outcome routines, reflexes, and similar operation units have a certain degree of autonomy when they execute their planned activities. Once they start to execute, they would continue according to their original plan until they reach their goal. However, the system must have means to intervene in the execution of planned activities. One reason is that two or more activities may be initiated at the same time, and they may need to use system's resources that can be used only by one plan at a time. The Brain Operation Supervisor (BOS) is a unit of the model whose responsibility is to coordinate the activities of plans that need to use such resources. The BOS can enable or disable the execution of activity plans and thus control their scheduling and prevent conflicts in using restricted resources. The BOS can also intervene in the ongoing operation of activity plans because of another important reason. At their inception, plans may not be able to take into consideration all the possible circumstances that could exist at the time of their execution. Consequently, that activity or its expected outcome may be in conflict with other ongoing operations or situations. In such cases, the BOS detects the conflict and intervenes. The BOS then would have four general options. First, it could terminate a controversial activity, thus eliminating the conflict. Second, it could allow the controversial activities to continue according to their original plans, so that the system 'absorbs' the consequences of the conflicts. Third, it could instruct a controversial activity to modify its plan, so that it might achieve its original goal without causing conflicts. Fourth, it could reschedule activities, if the conflict between them is due to their timing.

Circuitry and operation of a BOS

In order to effectively intervene in a planned activity, the BOS should be able to exert its influence, if possible, before that activity has been actually carried out. Two strategies could accomplish this requirement. In the first, all activities are disabled by default. An activity has to be enabled by the BOS before it is actually executed. The BOS enables an activity only if no conflict is anticipated. In the second strategy, all activities are enabled by default. An activity is disabled only if the BOS detects a conflict before its execution. The BOS has enough time to reach its decision, and to inhibit the execution of the controversial action before its start, if needed. In principle, the model can support these two strategies. In the following, it will be assumed that the BOS has the required capability, without specifying the details of the involved hardware design.

A conflict that requires a BOS intervention is caused by at least two activity plans, or an activity plan and a conflicting information entity. Figure 7.10 illustrates the relationships between the sub-units of a BOS and those of a controversial activity plan.

The operations of a triggered plan are coordinated by its plan-controller (figure 7.10). It activates the action sub-unit, and if needed, sets the traps for the goals. Planned activities are represented by their firing nodes at the action sub-unit. Those activities, though, may conflict ongoing activities outside of the unit. In such cases, the firing node at the action sub-unit together with its conflicting node outside of the unit will trigger the conflict detector of the BOS, which will trigger the BOS.

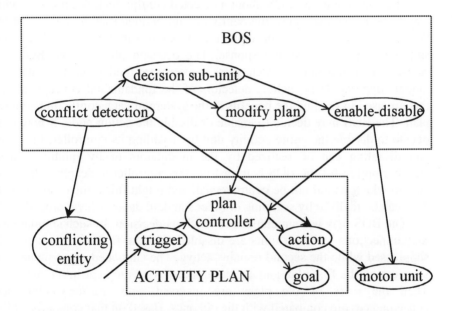

Figure 7.10: The relationships between the sub-units of the BOS and an activity plan. Thin arrowheads indicate direction of information flow.

Firing nodes of the action sub-unit may contribute to several types of conflicts. One type occurs when two nodes are attempting to set one motor-unit into two mutually exclusive states. For example, two nodes that are attempting to set the same motor-unit in relaxed and in contracted states, at the same time, are in conflict. This fundamental conflict is at the roots of broader conflicting motor-plans. For example, plans to walk forward and to walk backwards at the same time are conflicting, because they include conflicting instructions to some of their basic motor-units.

Another type of conflicts occurs when a situation associated with an action plan is conflicting an ongoing state or activity. For example, the action-plan to eat a sumptuous cake has an associated outcome that is conflicting an ongoing plan to be on a low calorie diet. An intervention of the BOS will decide which plan should be realized. A firing action-node can activate its associated node through any of the standard mechanisms that the model supports, such as completion, or a sequence of associations.

The message to the BOS about a detected conflict includes markers with which the nodes that cause the conflict could be identified and accessed by the BOS. That message prompts the decision sub-unit to evaluate the situation and to choose a response. The decision plans of the BOS are composed of fundamental detectors, constructors, and projectors that the model supports. They include detectors of the fundamental concept 'more' that are used in grading the benefits to the system of each conflicting activity plan. The BOS may decide to enable or disable the action node. It may also decide to disable the entire activity unit by disabling its controller. Enabling and disabling can be realized by the modulators or by inhibitory ties. Another option for the BOS is to instruct the controller to search a different action, which would not be controversial, and might fulfill the original goal. This can be realized by scanning or other standard data-retrieval procedures.

The BOS may use simulations to reach its decision. In such simulations, the connections to motor-units are disabled, and the first activation plan is suppressed while the second remains active. The simulated consequences of suppressing the first plan and executing the second are kept in the memory. Then the roles of the plans are reversed, and the new simulated consequences are compared with the old ones. Based on that comparison, the decision sub-unit may weigh the expected consequences of the various options, and choose the most appropriate one. The BOS may also simulate executing the two conflicting plans one after the other. If the simulation shows that the controversy would be resolved this way, the activity plans are scheduled accordingly, and executed.

A BOS may decide to require a controversial activity-plan to come up with a replacement action, which would not cause controversy. Actions that are co-exemplars of the controversial action are promising replacements. The activity plan could scan the memory for such exemplars. The BOS would then employ additional simulations to check the adequacy of any proposed replacement, and if an appropriate replacement is found, the BOS would stop the scanning and would enable the modified activity plan. If such simple scanning does not produce the desired result, retrieval of replacements according to other plans may be attempted.

Suppressing a plan may resolve an existing controversy, but may cause new ones. In addition, requiring an activation plan to search for non-controversial replacements may conflict with time constraints that the system has. In this sense, the BOS itself has action plans, whose activities may cause conflicts. The BOS can supervise its own action-plans, the same way that it supervises other plans.

The BOS is limited in its ability to resolve all the conflicts. Sometimes, conflicts are triggered by external conditions or by drives that cannot be resolved by the BOS. In addition, the BOS and the system may not be able to predict correctly all the outcomes of the activity plans, or the outcomes of their suppression. That may result in worsening a situation instead of improving it.

The BOS and consciousness

The brain can be in a number of consciousness states including the normal awake state, sleep, drug-induced states, meditation, hypnosis, and biofeedback. In each of these cases, only certain state-dependent memory records and computation units are accessible to manipulations by the brain.

The brain may be aware of the state in which it is found and of the nature of the ongoing processes. For example, when we are awake we are aware of that fact, and we are aware of ongoing thinking, sensory, and motor processes. Awareness and awareness features are fundamental concepts of the system, and as such, they are represented by nodes. Awareness detectors make awareness nodes fire according to the particular consciousness concepts that they have detected in the system. Awareness detectors can also participate in recording data in the memory. For example, a memory record of an event may include consciousness features, which have been provided by awareness detectors, such as "it was a sensory experience" or "it was a thought product".

In the normal awake state, a considerable amount of mental processes and the data that they use cannot be detected by awareness detectors. These constitute the unconscious part of the awake state. Other consciousness states have unconscious parts of their own. In general, conscious concepts of a state have connections to that state's awareness detectors and to other computation units. Unconscious concepts have no connections to consciousness detectors, but they have connections to other nodes and computation units.

The consciousness state of the system is affected in some cases by external factors, such as drugs, and in other cases by combinations of external and internal factors. In the model, the simulation program activates or deactivate the consciousness nodes that would have been activated or deactivated in the brain by drugs or other external factors. The simulation program also sets the connections between nodes, computation units, and consciousness detectors according to the situation in the simulated consciousness state.

There is some flexibility in the connections between nodes and awareness detectors. Existing connections may be changed temporarily or permanently, and new connections may be established.

Some of the nodes of a computation unit may be detectable by awareness detectors, while other nodes of the same unit may be undetectable. Often, we may be aware of the beginning and outcome of a process, but we are completely unaware of the steps leading from that beginning to the end.

Awareness detectors may have reciprocal connections with detectable nodes. By using these connections, an awareness detector may prime a quiet detectable node and make it more excitable to other stimuli.

Both conscious and unconscious processes take place in the system concurrently, and conflicts arising from any types of activity would trigger the BOS. When all conflicting activities are conscious, the system can be aware of how the BOS is resolving the situation. In various situations of stress, conflicts occur due to unconscious process or processes. The system may not be aware of the cause of the stress or the mechanisms that the BOS employs to alleviate it, but the system is aware of the stress itself.

The model assumes that in their execution, both conscious and unconscious processes employ the same fundamental procedures. The distinction between the two is due to them having or lacking connections with awareness detectors, but not due to the circuitry of the processes themselves. The BOS utilizes the same strategies to resolve problems that the system is aware of and unconscious problems that their presence may be inferred by the inexplicable stresses that they cause. These actions of the BOS affect the circuitry of the problematic activities and their connections to the rest of the system.

Conflicts that involve unconscious components play a central role in psychoanalytic theory, which recognizes a number of strategies that the system employs to resolve them. These include repression, rationalization, reaction-formation, displacement, and projection. The brain also uses the same strategies in resolving conscious problems. The following paragraphs illustrate how the BOS implements these strategies within the framework of the model.

Repression

When memory records of events that have stirred strong emotion are retrieved, they may invoke their associated emotions as a byproduct. Sometimes, those emotions are too hard for the system to relive. In order to prevent that undesired side effect, the system may use repression mechanisms, which make the record of the problematic event completely or partially irretrievable. Repression is also used to silence innate drives that have become stressing due to restrictions that the system has learned at some later stages. These include conflicts between innate id drives and their contradicting acquired super-ego edicts. For example, an aggressiveness drive aimed at a younger sibling would be repressed, because of the undesired feeling of parental disapproval, which most likely would follow its execution. The BOS, when triggered by such stressful feeling or controversy, can employ a number of repression mechanisms, which are supported by the model. The differences between the various repression mechanisms would determine the response of the system when an attempt is made to retrieve a repressed memory record or to activate a repressed drive.

Figure 7.11 illustrates as an example the memory record of an event that has to be repressed due to stressful feelings that it invokes. The event is the death of a dear friend, who died of in an accident. Whenever this memory is brought up, it invokes deep sadness that threatens the well being of the individual. The broader memory record consists of an event, whose parts are the concepts 'death', 'the friend', 'accident' and the ensuing feeling 'sadness'. (Not all the details of this data structure are shown). When the item-node that represents the entire occurrence is retrieved, it activates the trigger of the sensation of sadness, which is then felt by the individual. The system is aware of any existing concept that establishes connections to consciousness nodes, as described above. (Only some of the established connections to the consciousness nodes are shown).

Connections at three sited could be manipulated to accomplish repression. First (marked A in figure 7.11), between the part-nodes 'accident', 'death', 'the friend', and 'sadness' and their item-node, which represents the entire occurrence. Second (marked as B), between the item-node of the entire occurrence and the node that triggers the feeling of sadness. Third (marked as C), between the nodes of the memory record and the consciousness nodes.

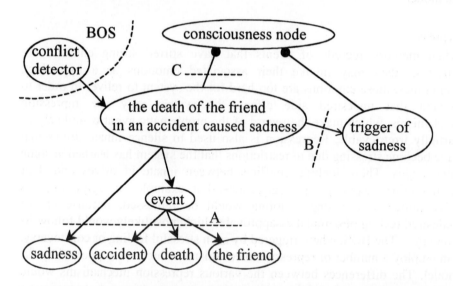

Figure 7.11: A memory record of an event that has to be repressed, and its relationships with other units of the system.

Usually, to be activated, item-nodes in memory records do not need all their part-nodes to fire. In this example, the firing of the part-node 'accident' or the part-node 'the friend'–by themselves–may activate the item-node of the entire event. This, in turn, would activate the trigger of the feeling of sadness. By weakening synaptic weights from those part-nodes to their item-node (marked A in figure 7.11), more firing part-nodes would be needed to trigger the item-node. In the extreme case, the synaptic weights may be reduced to a level that could not cause the activation of the item-node. That would completely repress the memory of the event and its unwanted effect, by making it irretrievable. Such weakening of weights happens sometimes even to benign memories due to aging, without an intervention of the BOS. We simply cannot recall events that happened a long time ago, when we get partial cues about them.

The second repression option would disconnect the node that triggers the feeling of sadness from the memory structure of the event (marked B in figure 7.11). That would eliminate the unwanted feeling, without affecting the memory records. It may be hard for to BOS to achieve that modification quickly, but sometimes it happens with time ("time is the best comforter"), or by habituation.

The third repression option relies on the interplay between consciousness-nodes and the nodes of which they are aware. In the last example, repression would amount to relegating the memory record of the entire event to unconsciousness. In the circuitry of figure 7.11, this kind of repression could materialize by disconnecting the class-exemplar connections between the consciousness-nodes and the memory node of the broader event (C in figure 7.11). However, disconnecting along C would still leave the 'sadness' node connected to the event node. If the connection between the two is strong enough, recalling the event will activate 'sadness'. If the connection between the two is not strong enough, and 'sadness' would normally need priming from the consciousness-node in order to be activated, disconnecting along C would preclude the firing of 'sadness'. This paradigm explains stresses that seep out to consciousness in spite of the repression. Such stresses will be generated if the connection between the node of the event and the sadness-trigger becomes strong enough to activate the sadness trigger without the help of the consciousness-node. Sadness will be felt, but the system will be unaware of its cause.

Repression mechanisms of drives are similar to repression of memory records. In such cases, the node that represents the drive plays the role of the offensive memory record when memories are repressed. For example, in repressing oedipal drives to get rid of the father, the node that represents that thought plays the same role as the node that represents the memory record of the event in figure 7.11. For at least some time, this repression eliminates the awareness of the offensive feeling that the drive would have caused. The drive itself, though, remains active unconsciously.

All these manipulations consist of basic operations of retrieval and weakening or trimming ties, which are supported by the model. The BOS applies them when information provided by the consciousness detectors indicates that the controversy is caused by retrieved memory records or by internal drives.

Noxious feelings or conflicts that are caused directly by external stimuli are detected and classified as such by consciousness detectors, which relay all that information to the BOS. It would not be wise to resolve these controversies by repression. Based upon the relayed information that the cause of the stress is external, the BOS would apply other appropriate strategies to resolve the problem. For example, a child would not repress fear that is caused by an external threat. Rather, the child would run away from the threat.

Rationalization

In rationalization, unacceptable thoughts or activity-plans are reinterpreted in an acceptable way, thus relieving the stress that they would have caused if left alone. For example, the stress-causing thought 'the dear friend died in an accident' is replaced by the comforting thought 'the dear friend who died in an accident lived long and full life'. In the model, the BOS is triggered by the stress, and identifies the concept that has caused it. Then, the BOS retrieves an item-node whose part-node is the problematic concept. That item-node should also trigger a positive feeling. This retrieved item-node replaces the problematic concept in the unacceptable thought or activity-plan, thus eliminating the stress. For example, the concept 'the dear friend who died in an accident lived long and full life' contains, as a part, the stress causing concept 'the dear friend died in an accident' (figure 7.12). In order to replace the second node with the first, the BOS reduces the synaptic weights from the problematic event to the node that triggers sadness (D in figure 7.12), and increases the weights between the event and the item-node that triggers a positive feeling (E in figure 7.12). If 'event' is now revoked, it would activate the item-node, representing the positive memory, by which it is contained. (For example, the cue 'an accident' would now revoke 'dear friend who died in an accident had full and long life'.) This, in turn, would trigger the positive feeling instead of the stressful one.

The general procedure that the BOS employs in rationalization consists of the following fundamental steps, which are supported by the model.

- Identify the node 'S' that triggers the stress-causing node ('S' is the node 'the death of the friend in an accident caused sadness' in this example).
- Identify the part-nodes 'P_1', 'P_2', etc. of 'S'. ('P_1' is 'event' and 'P_2' is 'sadness' in the example).
- Scan the item-nodes of the part-nodes 'P_1', 'P_2', etc. until a node 'G' that triggers good feeling is found ('G' in this case is 'dear friend who died in an accident had full and long life', which is the item-node of 'P_1').

- Reduce the weight between 'P₁' and 'S', and increase the weights between 'P₁' and 'G' (this affects connection D and E in figure 7.12).

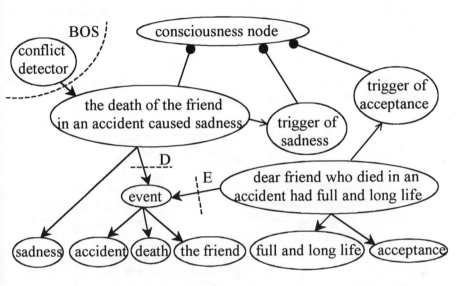

Figure 7.12: Example of nodes that are involved in a rationalization process.

Reaction formation

In reaction formation, a forbidden action that is a part of an information structure, and which causes an unpleasant consequence, is switched with an acceptable action. For example, instead of executing the impulse to hit her small brother, the older sister hugs and kisses him. The BOS has determined that pleasing the parents has more weight than getting satisfaction from hitting the brother. Based on that, hitting the brother, which is the less favorite plan, is modified in a reaction-formation process. Figure 7.13 illustrates the nodes and the activities that take place in this process of reaction-formation.

Once the BOS detects the conflict, it weighs the situation and decides which plan has to be modified. It identifies 'hit brother' as the controversial node that causes the conflict, and 'parental disapproval' as the affected feeling. The BOS employs the general reaction-formation routine, which consists of several standard retrieval requests. It can be formulated as:

- Retrieve a node 'A' that is a class-node of the controversial node (in this case, 'A' is 'interact with brother').
- Retrieve a node 'B', which is a mutually exclusive co-exemplar of the involved feeling (in this case, 'B' is 'parental approval').
- Retrieve a node that is an exemplar of 'A', of 'B', and of 'activity trigger' (in this case 'kiss and hug brother').

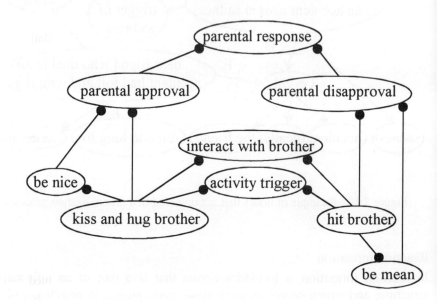

Figure 7.13: The memory structure that is used by the BOS to resolve the unacceptable impulse to hit the brother.

The execution of the modified action plan would probably result is gratification due to parental approval. However, some mixed feelings might remain–the impulse to hit the brother remains active and ungratified. To reduce these negative leftovers, the BOS may employ repression on that impulse, with various degrees of effectiveness.

Being exposed to other experiences in similar situations, such as 'share your toys with your brother', would eventually define the more abstract concepts of 'be nice' and 'be mean'. 'Be nice' would be associated at first with 'parental approval' and 'be mean' with 'parental disapproval'. These new concept-classes would then acquire exemplars that are not the result of experiences with the parents. The BOS would be able to use these new concepts in more mature reaction-formation processes.

Displacement

In displacement, an information structure contains an activity that is forbidden when applied to a specific individual, such as a sibling. The node of this individual is switched by another node, towards which the activity is not forbidden. Then, the activity is carried out. For example, the older sister, who cannot execute the urge to hit her little brother, spanks her doll instead. The operations that the BOS employs to accomplish displacement are very similar to those that accomplish rationalization, as mentioned above and as illustrated in figure 7.13. First, the BOS is triggered by the stress that the plan causes. The BOS then identifies the node 'S' that causes the stress ('S' is 'hit my little brother' in this example). Then, a part-node 'P' of 'S', which is also an exemplar of the class 'activities' is found ('P' is 'hit' in this case). An item-node 'G' that contains 'P' as its part-node, and which does not cause the negative side effects is found ('G' is 'hit the doll' in this case). Executing 'G' would send a feedback signal that the urge to hit was executed. Sometimes, that would quench the original urge. In addition, disapproval of the parents did not follow.

Projection

In certain situations, a scene that causes stress is represented by an information structure that contains nodes that represent the self and nodes that represent the cause of the stress. In what is called in psychoanalytical theory projection, the nodes that create the stress are cut off the structure and re-connected to a structure that represents another individual or entity. That eliminates or overshadows the original stress, and makes the other entity the target of the noxious feeling. In the model, the BOS can employ the fundamental 'switch' operation in order to execute this projection. (In the model, the term projection is used to describe a fundamental operation, which activates nodes in an arena to create a simulation of a real situation. This is different from 'projection' as used in psychology).

Two personas

The activity-plans and the states of the system can be divided into two main groups–conscious and unconscious. Each of these groups can get external stimulation, can use and manipulate memory records, has its goals, and can generate outputs for motor units. The same external stimulus or situation can trigger different conscious and unconscious activity plans. Each of those activity plans is wired to follow certain steps and to seek its own outcomes. In this respect, it may be said that the system consists of two competing **personas**, which are operating concurrently. These two personas attempt to control the same system, and because of that, conflicts between the two are inevitable. The system has a unit whose charge is to mediate the activities of the two personas. This basic and general view about the human psyche has been held in a variety of forms by many cultures and schools from ancient times to these days.

In the model, both conscious and unconscious activities are represented by the same hardware elements, and they employ the same operation rules. The BOS is the unit whose responsibility is to resolve stress causing and conflicting activity-plans. The BOS applies the same general strategies, such as those mentioned above, to resolve situations that are in pure conscious states, pure unconscious states, and in a mixture of the two. When the BOS resolves conflicts between two conscious activity plans, it is done in the open. The system is aware of both plans and of the give-and-take of the resolution process. When the BOS resolves conflicts that involve unconscious activity plans, the system cannot be aware of the exact nature of the conflict, and of the details of the compromise. The end product that the system gets may be an activity plan that has both conscious and unconscious parts. Such a unified activity plan is, in fact, a **pseudo-conscious activity plan.** When it is carried out, the system becomes aware of it and of its conscious steps. However, the system cannot be aware of its unconscious steps and their effect on the outcome. For example, if the brain has used rationalization as a stress avoiding mechanism, we might explain our motives for a certain action in one way, while unconscious forces that may have really drove that action remain hidden from us. The system may also have pseudo-conscious activity plans that are not the result of the merger of conflicting plans. In such cases, too, we may misinterpret the real drives behind our activities. Pseudo-conscious activity plans may be permanent or they may be put together for a given circumstance, and then disassembled.

In general, the system needs to update and to modify steps in its activity plans based upon its experiences. Apparently, it is simpler for the system to manipulate problematic nodes of conscious steps than to manipulate unconscious ones. Reciprocal connections from awareness detectors to activity units may be marking those conscious nodes, thus making them more accessible for modifications. Once the problematic nodes have been identified, the BOS can initiate processes that modify their circuitry, or construct other circuitry that bypasses or dominates the problematic segments. Making someone aware of unconscious segments in his or her activity plans is quite often the first step in treatments that alleviate stress and modify irrational behavior-patterns, which are detrimental to that individual.

The BOS and attention

In humans, attention is a heightened level of awareness. When stimuli or activity patterns are the center of the system's attention, the system is not only aware of them–the system also enhances their connections to certain detectors, projectors, and computation units. That facilitates the interaction between the attended stimuli and the rest of the system. For example, a student who is paying attention to his math teacher is not only aware of what she is saying. He is also enabling detectors, projectors, and computation units in his system to analyze what she is saying and to integrate the processed information in his system. Or, a high-wire-walker in a circus. He is not only aware of the wire and his feet. Sensors in his eyes, in his feet, and in his vestibular system, and computation units that control his posture are specifically primed and tuned to process all the vital incoming stimuli.

As long as the system is paying attention to certain stimuli, their representing nodes remain latched to units with which they exchange signals. Once the stimuli cease to be at the center of attention, their nodes are unlatched from those units. In many circumstances, it is the responsibility of the BOS to latch and unlatch stimuli-nodes to certain units, thus bringing the stimuli to the attention of the system. These latching and unlatching can be accomplished in a number of ways, depending on the circumstances. The system can pay attention to external stimuli for as long as they are present. All the system has to do is to lock its detectors on the stimuli. For example, by locking its gaze on its prey, a predator focuses its attention on it. In such cases, the BOS can employ feedback circuits to keep the gaze locked on the prey. In other processes, especially mental ones, the trigger of the process may be present, i.e. firing, for only a limited time. If the process has to proceed beyond that firing period, the BOS can latch the trigger's nodes and make them fire for as long as their firing is needed. When the latched nodes are unlatched, they are not attended any more, and the system can direct its attention to new stimuli. Normally, nodes that trigger attention should be unlatched when the computations that they call for are completed. In the model, latching and unlatching of a node can be accomplished by relying on core-activator hookups that the nodes have (figure 6.1), and on the standard processes of connecting and disconnecting nodes.

The model can represent two kinds of attention disorders. In attention deficit disorder, the nodes that are at the center of attention do not remain latched long enough, so that processes that depend on their firing cannot be completed. This can happen because the latching is not strong enough and fades away by itself, or because the BOS is hypersensitive to other ongoing activities that compete with the latched one, and switches the attention to them. In attention excess disorder, the attention sources remain unnecessarily latched after the computations have been completed, thus they cause the processes to repeat themselves for no apparent reason.

The model, determinism, and free will

The model presented here is deterministic. The state of the system at the end of any time interval is determined by its state at the beginning of that time interval and by the prevailing external conditions. The system's patterns of active nodes and the changes in its circuitry are derived based on deterministic activity rules of nodes and of computation units. This is true for any time interval, all the way back to the innate system. Thus, the state of the system and its actions at any given time are determined by its innate state, by its innate operation rules, and by its accumulated experiences–a combination of nature and nurture.

The basic laws of classical physics, as summarized by Newton's Laws and by Maxwell's equations, are deterministic. However, with the introduction of quantum physics around the first quarter of the twentieth century, it became clear that microscopic systems obey different laws, which are indeterministic in nature. Since then, the demarcation line between deterministic and quantum phenomena has been the subject of intensive research efforts. An apple falling to the ground can be described in a deterministic way, whereas the processes that cause its stem to break involve both classical and quantum effects. The brain and its function have also been the subject of such investigations. While many macroscopic activities of the brain demonstrate deterministic cause-effect relationships, other sub-cellular processes may obey the laws of quantum physics. At this time, the interplay between classical and quantum processes in the brain is still under study.

The model presented here uses deterministic laws to describe the operations of its nodes and networks. It seems that these deterministic laws can explain the relationships between operation at the neural level and the observed macroscopic behaviors of the brain. However, the nodes of the model could support probabilistic laws that would result from quantum processes of neurons and their sub-systems, if more information becomes available.

A question related to the deterministic nature of the system is the question of free will. It is said that when we choose the ice cream flavor that we like, vote for one party or another, lie or tell the truth, and so on, we are exercising 'free will'. The model can simulate these events. Because of its basic rules, all the activities that the model simulates are deterministic. A certain innate system that went through a certain sequence of life experiences will end up choosing strawberry ice cream. Next time, based on its accumulated experiences, that system may choose vanilla, but it is all done according to deterministic pre-set rules. So, does the model have 'free will'? If 'free will' is defined as a will that does not depend on pre-set mechanisms, the model does not have free will. Similarly, if all the biological processes at the neuron level and above are deterministic, there is neither free will in our own actions. Even if the neurons act according to probabilistic quantum laws, there is no free will in the system, because these probabilistic laws are pre-set. According to this view, there is no more free will in human actions than there is free will in a tree developing its roots and leaves.

It seems that what is referred to as "free will" in the examples above is a conscious decision process, in which various possible outcomes are being considered. This decision process may employ some unconscious mechanisms. These unconscious mechanisms, especially unconscious pre-set thinking processes, create the impression that the system has free will. The model possesses this kind of 'free will'.

Bibliography

Aleksander, I., *Impossible Minds: My Neurons, My Consciousness*. London: Imperial College Press, 1996

Aleksander, I., *Neurons and Symbols:The stuff That Mind Is Made Of*. London: Chapman & Hall, 1993

Arbib, M.A., [et al] (eds.), *The Handbook of Brain Theory and Neural Networks*. Cambridge, Mass.: MIT Press, c1995

Ballard, D.H., *An introduction to Natural Computation*. Cambridge, Mass.: The MIT Press, 1999

Baev, K.V., *Biological Neural Networks: The Hierarchical Concept of Brain Function*. Boston: Birkhauser Boston, 1998

Bechtel, W., Abrahamson, A. (eds.), *Connectionism and the Mind: Parallel Processing, Dynamics, and Evolution*. Cambridge, Mass.: Blackwell Publishers, 1999

Carlson, N.R., *Physiology of Behavior*. Boston: Allyn and Bacon, 1998

Churchland, P., Sejnowski, T.J., *The Computational Brain*. Cambridge, Mass.: The MIT Press, 1992

Conlan, R. (ed.), *States of Mind: New Discoveries About How Our Brains Make Us Who We Are*. Englewood Cliffs, NJ: Prentice Hall, 1999

Clark, A., *Associative Engines: Connectionism, Concepts, and Representational Change*. Cambridge, Mass.: The MIT Press, 1993

Elman, J.L. [el al], *Rethinking Innateness: A Connectionist Perspective on Development*. Cambridge, Mass.: The MIT Press, 1996

Gentner, D., Holyoak, K.J., Kokinov, B.K., (eds.), *The Analogical Mind*. Cambridge, Mass.: The MIT Press, 2001

Grainger, J., Jacobs, A.M., *Localist Connectionist Approaches to Human Cognition*. Mahwah, NJ: Lawrence Erlbaum Associates, 1998

Green, H.S., Triffet, T., *Sources of Consciousness: The Biophysical Computational Basis of Thought*. Singapore: World Scientific, 1997

Groves, P., Schlesinger, K., *Introduction to Biological Psychology*. Dubuque, Iowa: Wm. C. Brown, 1979

Harvey, R.L., *Neural Network Principles*. Englewood Cliffs, NJ: Prentice Hall, 1994

Holyoak, K.J., Thagard, P., *Mental Leaps: Analogy in Creative Thought*. Cambridge, Mass.: MIT Press, 1995

Horgan, T.E., Tienson, J., *Connectionism and the Philosophy of Psychology*. Cambridge, Mass.: The MIT Press, 1996

Jackson, S.A., *Connectionism and Meaning: From Truth Conditions to Weight Representations*. Norwood, NJ: Ablex Publishing Corporation, 1996

Levine, D.S., *Introduction to Neural and Cognitive Modeling*. Mahwah, NJ: Lawrence Erlbaum Associates, 2000

Metzinger, T. (ed.), *Neural Correlates of Consciusness: Empirical and Conceptual Questions*. Cambridge, Mass.: The MIT Press, 2000

Peretto, P., *An Introduction to the Modeling of Neural Networks*. Cambridge; New York: Cambridge University Press, 1992

Pickles, J.O., *An Introduction to the Physiology of Hearing*. London: Academic Press, 1988

Quinlan, P.T., *Connectionism and Psychology: A Psychological Perspective on New Connectionist Research*. Chicago: The University of Chicago Press, 1991

Rolls, E.T., Treves, A., *Neural Networks and Brain Function*. Oxford: Oxford University Press, 1998

Rosenzweig, M.R., Leiman, A.L., Breedlove, M.S., *Biological Psychology: An Introduction to Behavioral, Cognitive, and Clinical Neuroscience*. Sunderland, Mass.: Sinauer Associates, 1999

Rumelhart, D.E., McClelland, J.L., and the PDP Research Group, *Parallel Distributed Processing: Explorations in the Microstructure of Cognition, Vol 1&2*. Cambridge, Mass.: The MIT Press, 1986

Sigel, I.E., (ed.), *Development of Mental Representation: Theories and Applications*. Mahwah, NJ: Lawrence Erlbaum Associates, 1999

Stich, S.P., *Deconstructing the Mind*. Oxford: Oxford University Press, 1998

Tanenbaum, A.S., *Structured Computer Organization*. Englewood Cliffs, NJ: Prentice Hall, 1990

Thagard, P., *Mind: Introduction to Cognitive Science*. Cambridge, Mass.: MIT Press, 1996

Todd, P.M., Loy, G.D., (eds.), *Music and Connectionism*. Cambridge, Mass.: The MIT Press, 1991

Tunturi, A.R., (1952) A difference in the representation of auditori signals for the left and right ears in the iso-frequency contours of the right middle ectosylvian auditory cortex of the dog *Am. J. Physiol.* **168**, 712-727

Wasserman, P.D., *Advanced Methods in Neural Computing*. New York: Van Nostrand Reinhold, 1993

Wasserman, P.D., Oetzel, R.M., *NeuralSource: the Bibliographic Guide to Artificial Neural Networks*. New York : Van Nostrand Reinhold, 1990

Zurada, J.M., *Introduction to Artificial Neural Systems*. St. Paul: West, 1992

Index